Complementary and Alternative Medicine, Part I: Therapies

Editor

STEPHEN D. KRAU

NURSING CLINICS OF NORTH AMERICA

www.nursing.theclinics.com

Consulting Editor
STEPHEN D. KRAU

December 2020 • Volume 55 • Number 4

ELSEVIER

1600 John F. Kennedy Boulevard • Suite 1800 • Philadelphia, Pennsylvania, 19103-2899

http://www.theclinics.com

NURSING CLINICS OF NORTH AMERICA Volume 55, Number 4
December 2020 ISSN 0029-6465, ISBN-13: 978-0-323-76031-7

Editor: Kerry Holland
Developmental Editor: Casey Potter

Nursing Clinics of North America (ISSN 0029-6465) is published quarterly by Elsevier Inc., 360 Park Avenue South, New York, NY 10010-1710. Months of issue are March, June, September, and December. Periodicals postage paid at New York, NY and additional mailing offices. Subscription price per year is, $163.00 (US individuals), $518.00 (US institutions), $275.00 (international individuals), $631.00 (international institutions), $231.00 (Canadian individuals), $631.00 (Canadian institutions), $100.00 (US and Canadian students), and $135.00 (international students). To receive student/resident rate, orders must be accompanied by name of affiliated institution, date of term, and the signature of program/residency coordinator on institution letterhead. Orders will be billed at individual rate until proof of status is received. Foreign air speed delivery is included in all *Clinics* subscription prices. All prices are subject to change without notice. **POSTMASTER:** Send address changes to *Nursing Clinics*, Elsevier Health Sciences Division, Subscription Customer Service, 3251 Riverport Lane, Maryland Heights, MO 63043. **Customer Service: Telephone: 1-800-654-2452** (U.S. and Canada); **1-314-447-8871 (outside U.S. and Canada). Fax: 1-314-447-8029. E-mail: journalscustomerservice-usa@ elsevier.com** (for print support) and **journalsonlinesupport-usa@elsevier.com** (for online support).

Nursing Clinics of North America is covered in *EMBASE/Excerpta Medica, MEDLINE/PubMed (Index Medicus), Social Sciences Citation Index, Current Contents, ASCA, Cumulative Index to Nursing, RNdex Top 100,* and Allied Health Literature and International Nursing Index (INI).

Contributors

CONSULTING EDITOR

STEPHEN D. KRAU, PhD, RN, CNE
Associate Professor (Ret), Vanderbilt University School of Nursing, Nashville, Tennessee

EDITOR

STEPHEN D. KRAU, PhD, RN, CNE
Associate Professor (Ret), Vanderbilt University School of Nursing, Nashville, Tennessee

AUTHORS

STACEY G. BROWNING, DNP, MSN, RN
Assistant Professor of Nursing, Whitson-Hester School of Nursing, Tennessee Technological University, Cookeville, Tennessee

ELIZABETH BORG CARD, MSN, APRN, FNP-BC, CPAN, CCRP, FASPAN
Nursing Research Consultant, Nursing Research Office, Vanderbilt University Medical Center, Nashville, Tennessee

PATRICIA ELIZABETH DAVIES HALL, DNP, APRN, WHNP-BC
Assistant Professor, Belmont University School of Nursing, Nashville, Tennessee

DEBORAH L. ELLISON, PhD, MSN, BSN
Professor of Nursing, Austin Peay State University, School of Nursing, Clarksville, Tennessee

ASHLEY J. FARRAR, BSN, RN
Mayo Clinic Hospital, Apheresis Department, Phoenix, Arizona

FRANCISCA C. FARRAR, EdD, MSN, RN
Austin Peay State University, School of Nursing, Clarksville, Tennessee

CINDY HUI-LIO, EdD
Movement Instructor, Osher Center for Integrative Medicine at Vanderbilt, Vanderbilt University Medical Center, Adjunct Assistant Professor, Blair School of Music, Vanderbilt University, Nashville, Tennessee

STEPHEN D. KRAU, PhD, RN, CNE
Associate Professor (Ret), Vanderbilt University School of Nursing, Nashville, Tennessee

KATHIE LIPINSKI, MSN, RN
Private Practice: Healing from the Heart NY

CYNTHIA K. MEYER, MSN, BSN
Assistant Professor of Nursing, Austin Peay State University, School of Nursing, Clarksville, Tennessee

LEIGH ANN McINNIS, PhD, FNP-BC, RN
Professor, School of Nursing, Middle Tennessee State University, Murfreesboro, Tennessee

SALLY M. MILLER, PhD, RN
Assistant Professor of Nursing, Vanderbilt University School of Nursing, Nashville, Tennessee

ANGELA MOREHEAD, DNP, FNP-BC, RN
Assistant Professor, School of Nursing, Middle Tennessee State University, Murfreesboro, Tennessee

MELANIE HALL MORRIS, PhD, APRN, WHNP-BC, CCE
Assistant Professor, Vanderbilt University School of Nursing, Nashville, Tennessee

GARRETT SALMON, DNP, RN, CRNA, APN
Assistant Professor, School of Nursing, Middle Tennessee State University, Murfreesboro, Tennessee

RUTH E. TAYLOR-PILIAE, PhD, RN, FAHA, FAAN
Associate Professor, Nursing, University of Arizona College of Nursing, Tucson, Arizona

CLARE THOMSON-SMITH, DNP, JD, RN, FAANP
Assistant Professor of Nursing, Vanderbilt University School of Nursing, Nashville, Tennessee

JANE VAN DE VELDE, DNP, RN
Private Practice: The Reiki Share Project

RICHARD WATTERS, PhD, RN
Interim Director, Nursing and Health Care Leadership, Vanderbilt University School of Nursing, Nashville, Tennessee

Contents

insomnia. It is beneficial for preoperative anxiety, oncology, palliative care, hospice, and end of life. Essential oils can be dangerous and toxic, with some being flammable, causing skin dermatitis, being phototoxic with risk of a chemical burn, or causing oral toxicity or death. The article investigates history, supporting theories, guidelines, plant sources, safety, pathophysiologic responses, and clinical nursing aromatherapy. Recommendations for developing a best practice clinical nursing aromatherapy program are provided.

Health care organizations are responding to consumer demand by offering more complementary and integrative health services in inpatient, outpatient, and clinic settings. Nursing has long embraced energy-based modalities such as Reiki and has been at the forefront of introducing body, mind, and spirit healing practices into health care settings. This article describes how nurses can integrate Reiki into both their personal lives for self-care as well as their professional patient care practices. An overview of Reiki's integration into hospital systems is presented as well as Reiki's use with various patient populations. The status of Reiki research is discussed.

More Americans are embracing complementary and integrative healing modalities such as Reiki to enhance the efficacy of allopathic medicine. It is important that nurses and other health care professionals be knowledgeable about these modalities. Reiki is a wellness practice that offers whole-person healing of body, mind, and spirit. The study of Reiki offers nurses an opportunity to care for themselves as well as create an optimal healing environment for their patients. This article offer nurses a comprehensive overview of the system of Reiki; it includes the core elements of Reiki, its history, Reiki training, and examples of its applications.

The efficacy of using complementary and alternative medicine (CAM) is supported by the literature to decrease preoperative anxiety, postoperative pain and opioid requirements, as well as nausea and vomiting and to improve severity of headaches and increase wound healing. Nursing care includes interventions using CAs for treatment of a range of patient needs. Being supportive while educating parents and patients demonstrates altruism, which also is beneficial for improving health outcomes with CAM.

Evidence supports exercise as a first-line option for many chronic diseases. Although recommendations suggest 150 to 300 minutes a week of moderate-intensity or 75 to 150 minutes a week of vigorous-intensity aerobic activity, replacing sedentary behaviors with light-intensity activities reduces risks of all-cause mortality, and cardiovascular disease (CVD) mortality and incidence of CVD and type 2 diabetes mellitus. Exercise has positive effects on brain function, cognition, and depressive symptoms. Based on such evidence, health care providers should incorporate evaluation of physical activity into patient care. Patients should be evaluated for readiness and ability to exercise and encouraged to increase activity level.

Stacey G. Browning, Richard Watters, and Clare Thomson-Smith

This pilot study investigated the association between patient-specific, therapeutic music listening as a nursing intervention for mechanically ventilated patients, and the proportion of time those patients were considered to have intensive care unit delirium. The pilot study used the person-centered nursing framework as its theoretic foundation. Findings from an intimate prospective cohort design encourage an expanded look at potential benefits of therapeutic music listening in large, multisite, randomized clinical trials. Research and practice implications are discussed.

Angela Morehead and Garrett Salmon

Nausea and vomiting are complex symptoms related to many disease processes. With many pharmacologic interventions noted to have adverse effects, many patients are turning to alternative therapies, including acupuncture and acupressure. Their efficacy has been proven for nausea and vomiting related to pregnancy, in patients receiving chemotherapy, and in postoperative, pediatric, and female patients. There are minimal to no side effects with the use of acupuncture and acupressure for the treatment of nausea and vomiting. Providers should be encouraged to discuss the efficacy, benefits, and side-effect profile of acupuncture and acupressure with patients who suffer from nausea and vomiting.

Sally M. Miller, Cindy Hui-Lio, and Ruth E. Taylor-Piliae

Tai chi is an ancient Chinese internal martial art that has increased in popularity across the United States over the past 2 decades. Tai chi combines gentle physical movement, mental imagery, and natural, relaxed breathing. There is increasing scientific evidence showing the impact of tai chi exercise on multifaceted areas of health and well-being, including positive effects on cognition, depression, anxiety, sleep, cardiovascular health, and fall prevention. A review of the health benefits of tai chi exercise is presented, as well as recommendations for nurses seeking to answer patient questions about tai chi.

NURSING CLINICS OF
NORTH AMERICA

SERIES OF RELATED INTEREST

Critical Care Nursing Clinics of North America
https://www.ccnursing.theclinics.com/
Advances in Family Practice Nursing
http://www.advancesinfamilypracticenursing.com/

THE CLINICS ARE AVAILABLE ONLINE!
Access your subscription at:
www.theclinics.com

Preface

Complementary Interventions in the "New Normal?"

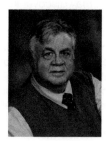

Stephen D. Krau, PhD, RN, CNE
Editor

The articles of this issue of *Nursing Clinics of North America* on Complementary and Alternative Medicine, Part I: Therapies were begun before the COVID-19 pandemic but were written during the pandemic. As such, some of the information warrants updating when describing how these interventions should be put into practice. It is important to follow the Centers for Disease Control and Prevention (CDC) Guidelines as well as any local, state, or regional guidelines. As mutable and different as these guidelines are, it would have been impossible to keep up with the standards during the development and publication of this issue. It is recommended that before implementing interventions, you check with your local officials for methods in which the current guidelines and recommendations should be implemented. We have many new standards in our nursing practice as a result of the pandemic. We also have many new standards in some areas as well, such as "social distancing," the use of gloves, and the wearing of masks to name a few. For optimal safety, please refer to your local agencies, to the CDC, and to organizations devoted to these specific interventions for the safest practice.

This issue was not designed to be an instruction manual in these interventions, although some articles have helpful information about how to begin some of these interventions. Many of the patients for whom we care utilize alternative therapies on a regular basis. A recent study by Taylor and colleagues[1] interviewed US veterans for their use of Complementary and Integrative Health (CIH) practices. The Veteran's Health Administration is the largest health care system in the United States. The subjects consisted of 530,216 veterans with chronic musculoskeletal pain. More than one-fourth (27%) of younger veterans with chronic musculoskeletal pain used any CIH therapy. It was found that 15% used meditation, 7% used yoga, 6% had engaged in acupuncture, 5% had engaged in chiropractic interventions, 4% used guided imagery, 3% used biofeedback, 2% had used tai chi, while massage was a method used by 2%,

Nurs Clin N Am 55 (2020) ix–x
https://doi.org/10.1016/j.cnur.2020.09.001
0029-6465/20/© 2020 Published by Elsevier Inc.

and 0.2% had engaged in in hypnosis.[1] The use of CIH therapies has increased tremendously over the last decade, and many health care organizations suggest variant alternative therapies in reducing pain, due to the overdependence on pharmacologic interventions for reducing pain.

As the use of complementary and alternative interventions increases in the United States, it is not unusual for nurses in practice to encounter patients who have used these interventions for any number of reasons. This issue of *Nursing Clinics of North America* introduces some of the many interventions that nurses may discover in their patients' histories. It is important to more fully understand the patient's health care needs, beliefs, and thoughts to better grasp the patient's trajectory. As part of this understanding, it is crucial to have some rudimentary knowledge of these interventions. This knowledge will enhance the nurse's comprehension of the patient's perception of health, their focus, thereby improving the link between the patient and the caregiver.

These articles are not a complete inventory of alternative therapies by any means, and this is also not a "how-to" issue; our goal is to familiarize the nurse with some alternative therapies of which the nurse may be unaware or not understand. There are organizations and certification programs for many of these alternative therapies that provide health care providers with knowledge and skills to become experts in these interventions, should one decide to pursue a specific intervention further. With the growing number of persons using these therapies, the purpose of this issue is to introduce the nurse to the basic ideas, principles, methods, and potential outcomes for these interventions. In March 2021, Part II will publish and address herbal supplements and vitamins, and I invite you to read both issues for a greater understanding of alternative and complementary medicine.

Stephen D. Krau, PhD, RN, CNE
Vanderbilt University School of Nursing
6809 Highland Park Drive
Nashville, TN 37205, USA

E-mail address:
sdkrau@outlook.com

REFERENCE

1. Taylor SL, Herman PM, Marshall NJ, et al. Use of complementary and integrated health: a retrospective analysis of US veterans with chronic musculoskeletal pain nationally. J Altern Complement Med 2019;25(1):32–9.

Presence and Therapeutic Listening

Deborah L. Ellison, PhD, MSN, BSN*, Cynthia K. Meyer, MSN, BSN

KEYWORDS

- Presence • Nursing presence • Therapeutic listening • Therapeutic relationship
- Nurse-patient relationship

KEY POINTS

- Presence and therapeutic listening are 2 critical elements in any complementary therapies used to develop a therapeutic nurse-patient relationship.
- Presence can affect patient outcomes by decreasing stress and anxiety, increasing safety and recovery, and producing an overall increase in patient satisfaction.
- Patient outcomes influenced by therapeutic listening include psychological benefits, promoting healing and recovery, and increasing quality of life and patient satisfaction.

INTRODUCTION

Complementary therapies have become widely known and used in Western health care because they play a key role in promoting healing, comfort, and care worldwide. Two therapies, presence and communication, are critical elements in the implementation of any of the complementary therapies.[1] Creating optimal health and/or healing environments with the implementation of complementary therapies, such as presence and therapeutic listening, is not limited by the environment or population.

The nurse-patient relationship, which is built on mutual trust and respect, is an important part of the nursing process. Trust is considered one of the most valuable concepts of communication and is directly related to effective communication, which is a major determinant of patient satisfaction.[2,3] Communication breakdown continues to be a problem within health care.[3] Building the nurse-patient relationship can be a difficult endeavor because of the numerous demands placed on nurses, and they must find a way to make patients feel valued and heard.

Healthy therapeutic nurse-patient relationships enhance wholeness and healing: they are key to effective health promotion.[4] Nurses must be able to incorporate the skills, knowledge, and attitude that allows the nurse-patient relationships to meet the patient where they are and build to a therapeutic relationship to implement

Austin Peay State University, School of Nursing, 601 College Street, Clarksville, TN 37043, USA
* Corresponding author.
E-mail address: ellisond@apsu.edu

Nurs Clin N Am 55 (2020) 457–465
https://doi.org/10.1016/j.cnur.2020.06.012   nursing.theclinics.com

presence and therapeutic listening. This article discuss the nurse's role in facilitating complementary therapies of presence and therapeutic listening, barriers encountered, and the techniques to be used. It also discusses the impact that using presence and therapeutic listening has on patient outcomes.

PRESENCE

Nursing presence is a complex concept that has not been well delineated in the nursing literature; nevertheless, despite the lack of clarity, it is central to concepts of caring and to behaviors such as listening and touch.[5] Nursing presence is both tangible and obscure at the same time. Therapeutic nursing presence shows caring, empathy, and connection, qualities required to build rapport and trust between nurse and patient.[4] Nursing presence is considered to be an essential state of holistic nursing as well as a core competency in contemporary nursing.[4] The concept of presence varies according to people's personal history of belief, sensory experience, and truths.[4,6]

DEFINITION

Nursing presence has been described as the art of nursing and is characterized as the "intentional use of self by the nurse who enters a reciprocal relationship with the patient, from an existential view."[7] Bright[5] (2015) described nursing presence as a "humanitarian quality of relating to a patient that is known to have powerful and positive implications for both nurse and patient." Mohammadipour and colleagues[8] (2017) provide an operational definition of nursing presence: "nursing presence is a concept that occurs via nurse-patient interactions within the health experience manifested through nurse's desire to begin interacting with patients, active listening, eye contact, calm speech, empathy, and subsequently accountable encounter."

NURSE'S ROLE

The concept of presence has long had roots in nursing, going back to Florence Nightingale, during the Crimean War, where she was known for establishing a nursing presence at the bedside of soldiers. Nightingale delivered compassion and care by dressing wounds, writing letters to soldiers' wives and mothers, and cared for the dying with a healing presence. This healing presence was attributed to her calm voice, warm smile, and gentle touch, which conveyed hope and trust. Nursing presence remains of interest to nursing scholars to this day. Patricia Benner[9] was essential in developing the concept of presence in contemporary nursing. Benner,[9] through her work:

1. Explained that nurses were trained to believe they were most effective by doing for the patient, not understanding that being with the patient could be as therapeutic
2. Designated the verb presencing as one of the 8 competencies of the helping role of the nurse
3. Explained that professional maturity, either innately or with experience, permits nurses to immerse themselves in a more meaningful exchange[9]

Benner[9] (1984) describes the expert nurse as one that can show the quality of presence. This work all lays the foundation for professional nurses now to be trained and skilled to provide nursing presence in nurse-patient relationships and to identify the value they provide to patient outcomes.[9]

In the nurse's role, nurses must be able to provide the physical, psychological, and spiritual presence, meeting the patients where they are for positive patient outcomes. If nursing presence is implemented correctly, the shared moments between the patient and nurse via relational connection facilitate participation with the patients and therefore enhance the nurse's ability to provide patient-centered care.[6,8]

NURSING BEHAVIORS

Nursing behaviors assisting in providing a positive nursing presence include:

- Using smiling
- Positive energy
- Holding silence with a patient
- Active listening
- Nurse's desire to begin interacting with patients
- Eye contact
- Calm speech
- Empathy[6,8,10]

There are also techniques that can be used by nurses that patients could view as providing a presence, which include:

- Mindfulness mediation
- Breathing techniques
- Guided imagery[6,8,10]

Although these subtle behaviors seem to be those that all nurses would use in any caring patient relationship, there is a more comprehensive nature of nursing presence that sets it apart from caring.[6] Nursing presence is not to change or intervene but to bear witness to the patient experiences in a nonjudgmental manner.[8,10]

BARRIERS

Many barriers prevent professional nurses from practicing with the intent of presence or using presence as an intervention with their patients. Modern nursing practice occurs in a system heavily influenced by protocols, standards of practice, staff shortages, equipment (technical, new, or shortage), lack of supportive environments, and endless lists of tasks to be accomplished.[5,6] Additional barriers include:

- Time
- Acuity of patients
- Training of nurses
- Technology
- Landscape of health care
- Willingness of patients
- Telehealth advances in health care

As the landscape of health care changes from acute care settings to population health in the community, nursing roles and expectations change. There are fewer nurses and higher-acuity patients in the acute care settings, which prevents nurses from always facilitating meaningful connections with patients. Technological advances in health care and communication have dramatically altered the landscape of caring in contemporary nursing practice in both acute care and community settings.[11] As already discussed, novice nurse may not have the maturity or experience to implement nursing presence in their practices. Health care has moved to virtual/

distance environments, and telehealth assessments can prevent nurses from maintaining a physical nursing presence with their patients along with making a personal connection with them.

THERAPEUTIC LISTENING

Therapeutic listening is one of the many tools nurses can use to help build the trust and respect that are needed. Therapeutic listening can convey empathy and confirm personal experience.[12] It can also facilitate growth and help convey warmth, empathy, and genuineness, qualities that are needed for growth.[12,13] Therapeutic listening can result in positive patient outcomes by reducing uncertainty, being perceived as trustworthy, friendly, and understanding.[12] Also, nurses who possess good listening skills can produce more satisfying interactions between patients and their physicians.[12] Therapeutic listening can also produce a sense of safety and understanding.[14] When therapeutic listening is achieved and the therapeutic relationship forms, effective communication can take place, leading to improvements in patient satisfaction, treatment adherence, quality of life, and anxiety and depression.[15]

DEFINITION

Listening, simply defined, means hearing or giving attention with the ear, but therapeutic listening goes far beyond and encompasses the art of being present, being alert to verbal and nonverbal cues, conveying warmth, and conveying an interest in the patient's current state.[16] Therapeutic listening can be defined as "an interpersonal, confirmation process involving all the senses in which the therapist attends with empathy to the client's verbal and nonverbal messages to facilitate the understanding, synthesis, and interpretation of the client's situation."[13] It can also be defined as a "method of responding to others to encourage better communication and cleared understanding of personal concerns."[17] For nursing, this is an important intervention that can be used to improve patient outcomes.

NURSE'S ROLE

The nurse's role in using therapeutic listening is to help facilitate and maintain the supportive, therapeutic relationship. It sounds simple but it takes work on the part of the nurse because therapeutic listening is a dynamic process that includes empathic responding with words and actions.[18] Nurses must be present and attentive to both the verbal and nonverbal communication that occurs within the interaction. Certain cues, such as facial expressions or tone of voice, are equally important as what is said. Nonverbal cues are presented in **Table 1**. Nurses must be alert for congruence between the verbal and nonverbal communication, because mixed messages may require reflection or validation to ensure that the message is clearly understood.[19] Cultural norms are an essential component of communication that should always be considered when interacting. For example, tone and pitch, facial expressions, and closeness when communicating can depend on cultural norms.[13,19]

There are other qualities that nurses can possess that lend themselves to therapeutic listening. These qualities help establish the trust and respect needed to ensure that the therapeutic relationship is established. Not every patient encounter requires therapeutic listening, but nurses must be prepared in any case. The following qualities are useful and **Table 2** discusses them in depth:

- Presence
- Self-awareness

Table 1
Nonverbal cues

Behavior	Possible Cues	Possible Meanings
Facial expressions	• Frowns • Smiles • Raised eyebrows • Grimacing	• Happiness • Sadness • Anger • Fear • Can be influenced by culture
Gaze and eye contact	• Intimidating gaze • Lowering brows • Avoidance of eye contact	• Respect • Lack of interest • Upsetting
Gesture and body movement	• Posture • Hand movements • Body movements • Gait/pacing • Head nodding • Touch	• Interest or lack thereof • Openness • Gestures can have different culture meanings
Spatial behavior	• Closeness of others	
Physical appearance	• Clothing • Grooming Hygiene	• Lack of interest • Energy

Data from Watanuki S, Tracy MF, Lindquist R. Therapeutic listening. In: Watanuki S, Tracy MF, Lindquist R, ed. Complementary & alternative therapies in nursing. 7th ed. New York: Springer; 2014: 39-50 and Varcarolis EM. Communication and the clinical interview. In: Halter MJ, ed. *Foundations of psychiatric mental health nursing.* 7th ed. Missouri: Elsevier; 2014: 147-164.

- Compassion
- Empathy
- Respect and understanding

BARRIERS

Nurses realize the importance of therapeutic listening and effective communication but often are faced with increased patient loads and list of tasks that take away from important patient interactions. Barriers include:

- Time
- Tasks

Table 2
Useful qualities of therapeutic listening for nurses

Being present	• Sets the intent of being there to listen • Allows nurses to listen and detect verbal/nonverbal cues
Using self-awareness	• Understanding of nurse's own values and beliefs • Aware of limitations
Showing compassion	• Establishment of caring
Empathizing with experiences	• Establishment of a caring environment • Establishes nonjudgmental acceptance
Convey respect and understanding	• Establishes rapport

Data from Refs.[2,5,6,10]

- Opportunities
- Charting/paperwork
- Administrative roles[12]

These barriers can directly affect the patients' perceptions of care. Patients report wanting someone to sit down and talk, personal contact, and to feel like they are more than a task, and therapeutic listening is one way to achieve this.[7] Patients with cancer have expressed feeling being undervalued, disrespected, and feeling ignored when they are not heard, which in turn leads to poor communication, and can affect the nurse-patient relationship.[18]

SKILLS AND TECHNIQUES

There are numerous skills and techniques used to facilitate therapeutic listening. It takes time to master this skill because it requires being fully present and truly listening, all while maintaining eye contact, maintaining attentive body language, and deciphering the verbal and nonverbal cues of the patient.[1,6,11] Because of time constraints and other barriers mentioned earlier, nurses may become distracted and not adequately focus on what is being conveyed or may miss an incongruence between what is said and the accompanying nonverbal cues.[5] In this instance, clarifying is a technique that can be used to assist in verifying the interpretation of the message or to create clarity.[5] Being present or giving good attention can be achieved by making adequate eye contact, leaning slightly forward, and giving short responses such as "uh-huh," and in turn can make patients comfortable and more willing to talk.[5,6]

Other techniques are summarized in **Table 3**.

OUTCOMES OF PRESENCE AND THERAPEUTIC LISTENING

Presence and therapeutic listening have been shown to positively affect several patient outcomes. Several themes were evident in the literature when researching patient

Table 3 Therapeutic listening techniques	
Silence	• Can be supportive • Allows time to think and formulate response • Reduces leading questions and lets nurse focus on message
Accepting attitude	• Nonjudgmental acknowledgment that patient has been heard • Creates a safe environment
Clarifying statements	• Verify the message • Avoid "why" questions
Restating	• Establishment of a caring environment • Establishes nonjudgmental acceptance
Reflecting	• Encourages self-understanding by directing feelings and ideas back to patient • Encourages patients to think for themselves • Paraphrasing to check understanding
Summarizing	• Brings everything together • Allows for clarification of any misinterpreted information
Making observations	• Uses nonverbal clues to verify message if incongruence between verbal and nonverbal message

Data from Refs.[3,13,14,19–21]

outcomes from using nursing presence and therapeutic listening. The main themes included decrease in stress and anxiety, increase in safety and recovery, and overall increase in patient satisfaction.[22,23]

Psychological benefits were seen in women with postpartum depression, who reported a decreased rate of anxiety and depression after having someone listen to them.[17] Others reported nursing presence and listening reducing the stress and anxiety brought on by illness.[8,10,24] Some patients have noted the importance having nursing presence and listening has on gathering clinical data and the ability to choose appropriate interventions, because they think their input is often ignored.[24]

As patient outcomes continue to be researched, there are several identified potential patient outcomes that are starting to appear in the literature. There is potential for increased treatment compliance when patients feel their input has been heard and that they are part of the team.[24] This outcome could be anything from a decrease in falls and pressure ulcers to changes in behavior modification with diet and exercise.[22] For adults living in long-term care settings, nursing presence and therapeutic listening can potentially increase quality of life, feelings of satisfaction and being grateful, and feelings of being cared about.[25,26] Presence and listening have the potential to create conditions that promote healing and recovery while also strengthening the therapeutic relationship. Patients reported valuing being treated as a unique individual, valuing being respectfully attended to, and an increase in nursing listening and nurse courtesy.[7,27]

The following is an example of how, by implementing a few of the techniques and behaviors of presence and therapeutic listening, professional nurse can create an environment for a trusting nurse-patient relationship and improved patient outcomes.

Example of Nursing Presence and Therapeutic Listening

A 56-year-old woman with hypertension is in for a check-up after having her medications changed because of uncontrolled hypertension. On assessment, the client's blood pressure is 186/98 mm Hg.

The patient becomes upset and states, "I have too much going on right now. My husband has been laid off, and I am taking care of my elderly mother."

The nurse, putting everything down and turning and leaning toward the patient, calmly states: "Tell me more about what is going on."

Client: "I have so much going on. I am helping my husband look for a new job and I have to take my mother to all of her appointments. Money is tight. I keep forgetting to take my medication."

Nurse: "You are very busy and this is a stressful time."

Client: "Yes, and I want to get my blood pressure under control, but I can't seem to make it a priority. I am so overwhelmed."

The nurse nods and calmly states: "Can you take a couple of deep breaths for me and when you're ready [short pause] go on."

Client: "I don't know how to remember to take them! [Sigh] Do you think if I should set an alarm on my phone and see if that helps? Maybe that would be a good reminder to take my pills."

Nurse: "You said that you're stressed and very busy. It sounds like you are overwhelmed, but you seem to have found a solution you are willing to try that could help."

SUMMARY

Presence and therapeutic listening are 2 complementary therapies that are incorporated into daily nursing practice. This article presents the nurse's role in facilitating complementary therapies of presence and therapeutic listening, barriers encountered, and the behaviors and techniques to be used. Also discussed was the impact that using presence and therapeutic listening has on patient outcomes. Nurses recognize the benefit and want time to be present and listen to what their patients have to say. These interventions have the potential to significantly alter patient' perceptions of care and improve patient outcomes. Presence and therapeutic listening are vital to developing a therapeutic nurse-patient relationship. This relationship is what drives positive patient outcomes and increases overall satisfaction and quality of care.

DISCLOSURE

Neither Dr D.L. Ellison or Mrs C.K. Myer has any commercial or financial conflicts of interest or any funding sources relevant to this article.

REFERENCES

1. Lindquist R, Snyder M, Tracy MF. Complementary & alternative therapies in nursing. 7th edition. New York: Springer Publishing Company, LLC; 2014.
2. Grover SM. Shaping effective communication skills and therapeutic relationships at work. AAOHN J 2005;53(4):177–82.
3. Stickley T, Freshwater D. The art of listening in the therapeutic relationship. Ment Health Pract 2006;9(5):12–8. Available at: https://journals.rcni.com/mental-health-practice/the-art-of-listening-in-the-therapeutic-relationship-mhp2006.02.9.5.12.c1899. Accessed April 2, 2020.
4. Boeck PR. Presence: a concept analysis. SAGE Open 2014. https://doi.org/10.1177/2158244014527990.
5. Bright AL. A Critical Hermeneutic Analysis of Presence in Nursing Practice." Humanities (2076-0787), vol. 4, no. 4, Dec. 2015, p. 958. EBSCOhost. Available at: http://search.ebscohost.com/login.aspx?direct=true&db=edb&AN=111965715&site=eds-live&scope=site. Accessed April 2, 2020.
6. Mohammadipour F, Atashzadeh-Shoorideh F, Parvizy S, et al. Concept development of 'nursing presence': application of schwartz-barcott and kim's hybrid model. Asian Nurs Res (Korean Soc Nurs Sci 2017;1:19.
7. Wendy B, Hansbrough, Georges Jane M. Validation of the presence of nursing scale using data triangulation. Nurs Res 2019. https://doi.org/10.1097/NNR.0000000000000381.
8. Mohammadipur F, Atashzadeh-Shoorideh F, Parvizy S, et al. Concept Development of Nursing presence": Application of Schwartz-Barcott and kim's hybrid model. Korean Society of Nursing Science Elsevier Korea; 2017. p. 1976-7. http://dxdoi.org/10.1016/j.anr.2017.
9. Benner PE. From novice to expert: excellence and power in clinical nursing practice. Menlo Park (CA): Addison-Wesley Pub. Co., Nursing Division; 1984.
10. du Plessis E. Presence: a step closer to spiritual care in nursing. Holist Nurs Pract 2016;30(1):47–53. Accessed February 9, 2020.
11. Grumme VS, Barry CD, Gordon SC, et al. On virtual presence. Adv Nurs Sci 2016; 39(1):48–59. Accessed February 9, 2020.
12. Weger H Jr, Bell GC, Minei EN, et al. The relative effectiveness of active listening in initial interactions. International Journal of Listening 2014;28(1):13–31. Available at: http://doi.org/10.1080/10904018.2013.813234. Accessed April 1, 2020.
13. Watanuki S, Tracy MF, Lindquist R. Therapeutic listening. In: Watanuki S, Tracy MF, Lindquist R, editors. Complementary & alternative therapies in nursing. 7th edition. New York: Springer; 2014. p. 39–50.

14. Bryant L. The art of active listening. Pract Nurse 2009;37(6):49–52.
15. Kornhaber R, Walsh K, Duff J, et al. Enhancing adult therapeutic interpersonal relationships in the acute health care setting: an integrative review. J Multidiscip Healthc 2016;9:537–46.
16. Listen. In: Merriam-Webster. 2020. Available at: https://www.merriam-webster.com/dictionary/listening. Accessed April 3, 2020.
17. Mesquita AC, Campos de Carvalho E. Therapeutic listening as a health intervention strategy: an integrative review. Rev Esc Enferm USP 2014;48(6):1123–31.
18. Nemec PB, Spagnolo AC, Soydan AS. Can you hear me now? Teaching listening skills. Psychiatr Rehabil J 2017;40(4):415–7.
19. Varcarolis EM. Communication and the clinical interview. In: Halter MJ, editor. Foundations of psychiatric mental health nursing. 7th edition. St Louis (MO): Elsevier; 2014. p. 147–64.
20. Jones A. The foundation of good nursing practice: effective communication. J Ren Nurs 2012;4(1):37–41.
21. Delaney KR, Shattell M, Johnson ME. Capturing the interpersonal process of psychiatric nurses: a model for engagement. Arch Psychiatr Nurs 2017;31:634–40.
22. Kostovich CT, Clementi PS. Nursing presence: putting the art of nursing back into hospitals orientation. J Nurses Prof Dev 2014;30:70–5.
23. Penque S, Kearney G. The Effect of Nursing Presence on Patient Satisfaction. Nurs Manage 2015;4:38. EBSCOhost, Available at: search.ebscohost.com/login.aspx?direct=true&db=edsgea&AN=edsgcl.410628509&site=eds-live&.scope=site.
24. Jagosh J, Boudreau JD, Steinert Y, et al. The importance of physician listening from the patients' perspective: enhancing diagnosis, healing, and the doctor-patient relationship. Patient Educ Couns 2011;85:369–74.
25. Jonas-Simpson C, Fisher A. The experience of being listened to: a qualitative study of older adults in long-term care settings. J Gerontol Nurs 2006;32(1):46–53.
26. An G-J, Jo K-K. The effect of a nursing program on reducing stress in older adults in two Korean nursing homes. Aust J Adv Nurs 2009;26:79–85.
27. Stockmann C. Presence in the nurse–client relationship: an integrative review. Int J Hum Caring 2018;22(2):49–64.

The Multiple Uses of Guided Imagery

Stephen D. Krau, PhD, RN, CNE

KEYWORDS

• Guided imagery • Visualization • Complimentary medicine intervention

KEY POINTS

• Guided imagery is a complimentary intervention that has been used for centuries.
• Guided imagery has multiple effects, including relaxation, stress reduction, anxiety reduction, immune system enhancement, and overall well-being.
• Guided imagery incorporates 5 main steps: assessing the issue, establishing a relaxed body position, using a focused breathing pattern, establishing a positive imagery environment, and beginning the "journey."

With the United States facing a so-called opioid epidemic, it is important to identify and use therapies that reduce pain but that do not involve pharmacologic interventions. There are a variety of nonpharmacologic interventions that not only have been shown to ameliorate pain, and the perception of pain, but that have been shown to help patients' mood, decrease anxiety, enhance relaxation, support behavior modification, and improve the immune system. One method that has shown all of these modifications is the use of imagery. It is common to have patients who have engaged in mental imagery for a variety of reasons, because imagery takes on many forms. As such, it is important to know how the patients have used imagery, the reasons they have used imagery, and the expected outcomes. Understanding this intervention improves the care nurses offer their patients, because it allows them to comprehend more about their patients and their patients' values and beliefs.

Imagery is a nonpharmacologic intervention that can accessed in a variable manner, and usually is inexpensive. There are a variety of methods that incorporate the use of imagery, but, regardless of the form, or name, the method typically involves the mental representation of a future situation, task, or event.[1] One of the more common forms of mental imagery is referred to as guided imagery. Guided imagery is sometimes referred to as guided meditation, visualization, mental rehearsal, or guided self-hypnosis. It can be as simple as a ski jumper's 10-second pause to consider the perfect ski jump and imagining how perfect it would feel to fly through the air and come to a perfect landing and slide. It can be more complicated to help individuals alter

Vanderbilt University School of Nursing, 6809 Highland Park Drive, Nashville, TN 37205, USA
E-mail address: sdkrau@outlook.com

Nurs Clin N Am 55 (2020) 467–474
https://doi.org/10.1016/j.cnur.2020.06.013
0029-6465/20/© 2020 Elsevier Inc. All rights reserved.
nursing.theclinics.com

behavior, or reduce anxiety and stress, by imagining positive interactions and scenarios to a real or potentially distasteful or anxiety-producing personal interaction.

GUIDED IMAGERY

Imagery is a technique that has been used in a variety of forms for centuries, even as far back as ancient Greek times. In the history of other cultures, the technique of guided imagery is a well-established therapeutic approach, as found in Chinese medicine and American Indian traditions. There are currently a variety of organizations that exist to help health care providers become imagery therapists, including certification programs in guided imagery.

Guided imagery is a mind-body technique that incorporates mental images to enhance an overall sense of well-being and to promote relaxation. In some cases, it involves the incorporation of visualization from direct imagery-based suggestion, or is the result of metaphor use and storytelling.[2] Guided imagery is based on the notion that the mind and the body are interrelated and can have bilateral interactions. As such, the brain is stimulated to envision an event in a positive and affirmative manner before the experience of the actual event. In essence, the individual is guided to develop an advantageous image mentally with a focus on the imagination to feel, see, hear, and smell the event as though it was real. It involves all of the senses, which is important because individuals learn differently and perceive differently; it is thought that only 55% of the population are primarily visually oriented, so the incorporation enriches the experience and the overall outcome that the individuals seek.

The individual's thoughts and imagination are focused and engaged toward a specific goal or outcome using a facilitator. The facilitator can be another person who is trained in guided imagery, or an audio tape or recording. Guided imagery can be used conjunctively with traditional interventions to specifically alleviate pain and/or to promote relaxation.[2] Through this process, individuals are mentally transported to a place where they feel safe and can be relaxed. The technique is easy to implement, not expensive, and not associated with adverse effects. Essentially, it is thought that the imagination of the individual is harnessed to overcome physiologic and psychological symptoms by the ability to send messages and information to the central nervous system to affect the body's physiologic processes.[2] Guided imagery is based on the principle of psychophysiology in that every thought results in a physiologic reaction, and a mental image invokes an associated emotion that connects the feeling state with the mind and body, which results in a physiologic change.[3]

GUIDED IMAGERY RELATED TO PAIN AND HEALING

One of the many benefits of guided imagery is targeted to a patient's healing and relief from pain. Because there is national concern about the opioid epidemic, modalities to alleviate pain adjuvant to pharmacologic solutions have helped bring to the forefront a focus of complimentary and integrative health (CIH) strategies, including the use of guided imagery. There are several theories related to the workings of guided imagery and how it affects pain and healing. One theory behind the process by which guided imagery affects pain and healing can be linked to the psychoneurological theory and the gate control theory.[4] It is postulated that, when a person creates an image, the cerebral cortex of the brain is in turn activated. As that image is held, the limbic system becomes activated, which in turn creates changes in the autonomic nervous system. According to the gate control theory, which remains controversial, the stimulation of the cerebral cortex caused by the image competes with pain stimuli, which closes the theoretic pain gate. This process occurs in conjunction with the secretion of neurotransmitters, which suppress pain transmission and support the inhibitory neurons in the secretion of natural opioids.[4] This theory is one theoretic hypothesis of how guided imagery works. This conjecture is difficult to support, as stated by King,[4] (2010) who conducted a thorough analysis of the effects of guided imagery on patients with cancer with pain. The inconsistencies among the studies in the analysis made it difficult to conclude that guided imagery should be recommended for all patients experiencing cancer pain.[4] The review consisted of small sample sizes, variations in the measurement of pain, different patient populations, and variations in guided imagery treatment times. Although the evidence is not strong or absolute, the analysis did conclude that guided imagery could be recommended as a potential aid in the relief of pain caused by cancer.

A controlled study by De Paolis and colleagues[5] (2019) had 104 randomized patients with advanced cancer using a combination of progressive muscle relaxation (PMR) and interactive guided imagery. Approximately one-third of patients with terminal cancer experience moderate to severe pain. These patients experience a myriad of emotions that affect psychological, affective, emotional, and spiritual aspects. It is also thought that these patients, as they become more preoccupied with their impending deaths, have catastrophic thoughts that have a tendency to amplify the perception of pain.[6] The purpose of guided imagery and PMR is thought to be to distract the patients from their perceptions of pain and physical deterioration, and to enhance their ability to control pain and, to some extent, their self-efficacy. The researchers had data showing that guided imagery had the ability to control pain and to improve the quality of life of patients with cancer and/or chronic pain associated with cancer.[7–14] This strong study of 104 randomized patients supported the efficacy of adjuvant PMR and guided imagery in alleviating pain distress in patients with terminal cancer.[5]

In an effort to address the opioid crisis, a group of researchers examined common CIH approaches in US veterans with chronic musculoskeletal pain.[15] The nation's largest integrated health care system has been a leader in increasingly offering CIH therapies.[15] It was found that more than 27% of younger veterans with chronic musculoskeletal pain used CIH, including meditation, yoga, acupuncture, biofeedback, tai chi, hypnosis, and massage. Many of the subjects thought that yoga was for girls.[15] The study revealed that 4% used guided imagery to control their pain. Of note in this study, younger men and African American men were less likely to engage in CIH therapies than older white patients. These findings are similar to the general population.[13]

GUIDED IMAGERY AND ITS IMPACT ON PAIN, ANXIETY, AND QUALITY OF SLEEP

A randomized 2-group experimental research design was used to study the effect of guided imagery on the pain, anxiety, and perceived quality of sleep of patients with fibromyalgia.[16] The study was supported by previous findings of another study showing that guided imagery improved overall quality of life.[17] The 2-group randomized study explored the impact of guided imagery using a program that was based on an audio program of relaxation guided imagery audiotapes. The intervention group had sessions on how to use the guided imagery audio program, and group discussions, and were asked to use the audio guided imagery CD at least 4 or 5 times per week over an 8-week period. The control group received 3 relaxation sessions of 1.5 hours, along with data collection.

At the beginning of the study, there were no significant differences between the two groups with regard to trait anxiety, state anxiety, sleep quality (except duration), pain at sensitive areas, or effects of fibromyalgia as measured by the Fibromyalgia Impact Questionnaire (FIQ).[16] The results of the study indicated that guided imagery relaxation in patients with fibromyalgia can be a favorable therapy when managing pain at tender points, anxiety, sleep, quality of life, and self-efficacy.[16]

GUIDED IMAGERY AND FOOD CRAVINGS AND CONSUMPTION

Guided imagery has also been studied as a method to reduce food cravings, and achieve behavioral modification of food consumption.[18] In 1 study, the investigators used guided imagery and cognitive defusion together with a study group of 127 women who reported experiencing at least 1 food craving per day. The participants were allocated to 3 groups. One group received cognitive defusion (n = 42), 1 received guided imagery (n = 39), and 1 served as the control group (n = 37).[18] Through their vigorous research process, the investigators discovered that cognitive defusion and guided imagery reduced the subjects' craving intensity and frequency, but these interventions also reduced craving-related food consumption.[18] There was no significant difference between guided imagery and cognitive defusion in reducing cravings or consumption.

GUIDED IMAGERY AND IMMUNE SYSTEM ENHANCEMENT

Trakhtenberg[19] (2008) conducted an extensive and critical review of the impact of guided imagery on the immune system. The review supports the use of guided imagery in the reduction of stress. In turn, reduction of stress enhances the immune system as measured in the literature primarily by white blood cell count. The author concludes

---

Box 1
The impact of guided imagery on the immune system

There is a relationship among guided imagery, stress and relaxation, and immune function.

Guided imagery as a relaxation intervention can reduce stress and allow the immune system to function more effectively.

Changes in immune system efficacy are correlated with either an increase or decrease in white blood cell count or with changes in neutrophil adherence.

Stress and relaxation may contribute to changes in the immune system when measured qualitatively by nature of neutrophil adherence, or quantitatively by white blood cell count.

Cell-specific imagery may predict which white blood cell category changes will occur.

An active cognitive exercise initiated in the beginning stages of guided imagery is associated with decreased neutrophil adherence.

Relaxation without an active imagery application is associated with increases in neutrophil adherence.

Decreases in white blood cell count occur only in early stages of guided imagery and/or relaxation interventions.

After 4 to 5 weeks of guided imagery and or relaxation, white blood cell counts increase.

Decreases and increases in white blood cell counts could be caused by the effect of margination, which means that the imagining training may be changing the movement of the white blood cells in the body, as opposed to the imagery sessions themselves and the white blood cell count overall not changing.

The change in white blood cell count may occur earlier in persons who present with a depressed white blood cell count and later in persons with normal white blood cell counts.

Adapted from Trakhtenberg, E. The effects of Guided Imagery on the Immune System: A Critical Review, *International Journal of Neuroscience,* (2008); 118:839-855 with permission.

that more long-term studies of guided imagery are needed to fully understand the impact of guided imagery on the immune system.[19] However, information gleaned from the review is extensive and has many implications for patient care. **Box 1** presents an overview of Trakhtenberg's[19] findings.

OVERVIEW OF GUIDED IMAGERY MECHANISM IN CRITICAL CARE

Although guided imagery is commonly seen in outpatient and noncritical in-patient settings, there are cases where guided imagery has been shown to be beneficial in critical care.[20] A review explored the effects of guided imagery on critical illnesses. The outcome measures seen in the review included pain, anxiety, hemodynamic measurements, stress neuropeptides, length of patient stay, sleep quality, inflammatory markers, patient satisfaction, and overall cost of care. The selection criteria allowed for 10 studies, which included 1391 critically ill patients. In any review there are limitations with inconsistent measurements, missing or incomplete data, or variations in the data used.

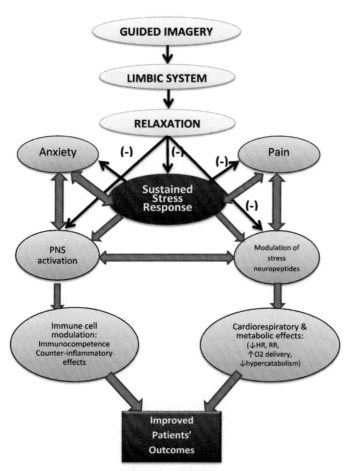

Fig. 1. Synthesis of mechanism involved in guided imagery effects. HR, heart rate; RR, respiration rate. (*From*: Hadjibalassi M, et al. The effect of guided imagery on physiological and psychological outcomes of adult ICU patients: A systematic literature review and methodological implications, *Aust Crit Care* (2018);31(2):73-86.)

The outcomes of the review were favorable in supporting guided imagery as an intervention in critical care. Effects were primarily seen in the reduction of pain, anxiety, and length of stays primarily in cardiovascular patients with moderate to high support.[20] Quality of sleep, patient satisfaction, and cost of care were difficult to support because of the limited number of studies that included these markers. The reviewers identify that there are other aspects related to critical care patients that could be included in future studies related to the impact of guided imagery on critically ill patients. For example, duration of mechanical respiration, rate of complications, stress neuropeptide levels, and immune measures warrant exploration.[20] The review lent itself to a depiction of the scheme of the proposed mechanisms of guided imagery with regard to critical illness (**Fig. 1**). Guided imagery acts early in the pathophysiologic cascade in which an exaggerated stress situation results in unfavorable effects in critical illness by activating the relaxation response. This response counterbalances the exaggerated stress response in the limbic system. It also activates the parasympathetic nervous system signaling and activating stress neuropeptides. Through these complex pathways, immune, cardiorespiratory, and metabolic responses are regulated, which results in improved patient outcomes.

STEPS USED IN GUIDED IMAGERY

This article presents an overview of guided imagery and the impact it has on patient care. There are variations in the process, as discussed, and, with advancing technology, the ability to access patients has become more efficient through telemedicine.

Table 1 Common steps to guided imagery	
Step 1: Assessing the problem	Establish the reason for the individual to engage in guided imagery. Determine whether the point is to reduce pain, create relaxation, reduce stress, enhance sleep, or reduce anxiety. Establish with the individual, or yourself, places that are considered "happy"
Step 2: Assume a relaxed position	Typically lying on the back with hands at the sides is a generic relaxation position. If a person finds this positioning painful, it is important to explore other options. Identify the position that the individual finds most comfortable for sleep. The use of a pillow or warm blanket is sometimes helpful
Step 3: Controlled breathing pattern	Once a comfortable position is established, the focus turns to breathing. Deep breathing alone has been shown to have numerous mental and health benefits. Breathing through the nose and out the mouth is recommended. Count up to 3 s while inhaling and 5 s while exhaling. Use an easy tempo for the individual and keep a focus on the breathing throughout the session
Steph 4: Create an imagery environment	At this juncture, create the environment that was discussed and decided on earlier to deepen the relaxation. Within this environment, incorporate all of individual's senses
Step 5: Begin the journey	Once the patient is relaxed and the imagined environment is created, it is then time to guide the experience. This guidance is contingent on the desired outcome of the session

Adapted from Integrative Pain Science Institute. 5 Steps to easing pain with guided imagery. https://www.integrativepainscienceinstitute.com/guided-imagery-5-steps/ Accessed 5/17/2020; with permission.

There are several associations that offer education, training, and certification to persons wish to become guided imagery therapists. For the elimination of pain, there are 5 common steps to conducting guided imagery. **Table 1** reviews those steps.

SUMMARY

Guided imagery is a therapeutic technique that has been used for centuries. As science and research have progressed, the efficacy of guided imagery has become better understood and has been used in practice with positive outcomes. Techniques vary because guided imagery can be done alone by individuals, with a guided imagery therapist in an individual session, in group sessions, or in remote sessions with the use of technology. With the further development of virtual reality technologies, the possibilities of guided imagery interventions become innumerable. Telemedicine is already a method of engaging a guided imagery therapist. Virtual technology has the capacity to help individuals create their safe places and virtually transport the individuals to those safe places. There remain many questions that warrant further exploration as they relate to patient outcomes. Research that standardizes measurements, methods, and controls will enhance the support of guided imagery.

REFERENCES

1. Conroy D, Hagger MS. Imagery interventions in health behavior: a meta-analysis. Health Psychol 2018;37(7):668–79.
2. Beizaee Y, Rejeh N, Heravi-Karimon M, et al. The effect of guided imagery on anxiety, depression and vital signs in patients on hemodialysis. Complement Ther Clin Prac 2018;33:184–90.
3. Jallo N, Ruiz RJ, Elswick RK, et al. Guided Imagery for stress and symptom management in pregnant African American women. Evid Based Complement Alternat Med 2014;840923. Available at: http://doi.org/10.1155/2014/840923. Accessed May 15, 2020.
4. King K. The review of the effects of guided imagery on cancer patients with pain. Complement Health Pract Rev 2010;15(2):98–107.
5. De Paolis G, Naccarato A, Cibelli F, et al. The effectiveness of progressive muscle relaxation and interactive guided imagery as a pain-reducing intervention in advanced cancer patients: A multicentre randomized controlled non-pharmacological trial. Complement Ther Clin Prac 2019;24:280–7.
6. Avy J. The impact of imagery on cognition and belief systems. Eur J Clin Hypn 2004;5:12–4.
7. Chen YL, Frances AJP. Relaxation and imagery for chronic, nonmalignant pain: effects on pain symptoms, quality of life, and mental health. Pain Manag Nurs 2010;11:159–68.
8. Sloman R. Relaxation and imagery for anxiety and depression control in community patients with advanced cancer. Cancer Nurs 2002;25:432–5.
9. Freeman L, Cohen L, Stewart M, et al. The experience of imagery as a post-treatment intervention in patients with breast cancer: program, process, and patient recommendations. Oncol Nurs Forum 2008;35:116–21.
10. Lewandowski WA. Patterning of pain and power with guided imagery. Nurs Sci Q 2004;17:233–41.
11. Mansky PJ, Wallerstedt DB. Complementary medicine in palliative care and cancer symptom management. Cancer J 2006;12(5):425–31.
12. Roffe J. A systematic review of guided imagery as an adjuvant cancer therapy. Psycho Oncol 2005;14:607–17.

13. Clarke TC, Black LI, Stussman BJ, et al. Trends in the use of complementary health approaches among adults: United States, 2002–2012. National Health Statistics Reports; No. 79. Hyattsville (MD): National Center for Health Statistics; 2015.

14. Downey L, Engelberg RA, Standish LJ, et al. Three lessons from a randomized trial of massage and meditation at end of Life: patient benefit, outcome measure selection, and design of trials with terminally ill patients. Am J Hosp Palliat Care 2009;26:246–53.

15. Taylor SL, Herman PM, Marshall NJ, et al. Use of complementary and integrated health: A retrospective analysis of U.S. Veterans with Chronic Musculoskeletal Pain Nationally. J Altern Complement Med 2019;25(1):32–9.

16. Onieva-Zafra MD, Parra-Fernandez ML, Fernandez-Martinez E. Benefits of a home treatment program using guided imagery relaxation based on audio recordings for people with fibromyalgia. Holist Nurs Pract 2019;33(2):111–20.

17. Luciano JV, D'Amico F, Cerda-Lafont M, et al. Cost-utility of cognitive behavioral therapy versus U.S. Food and Drug Administration recommended drugs and usual care in the treatment of patients with fibromyalgia: an economic evaluation alongside a 6-month randomized control trial. Arthritis Res Ther 2014;16(5):451. Available at: https://www.ncbi.nlm.nih.gov/pubmed/25270426. Accessed May 17, 2020.

18. Schumacher S, Kemps E, Tiggeman M. Cognitive defusion and guided imagery tasks reduce naturalistic food cravings and consumption. Appetite 2018;127: 393–9.

19. Trakhtenberg EC. The effects of guided imagery on the immune system: a critical review. Int J Neurosci 2008;118(6):839–55.

20. Hadjibalassi M, Lambrinou E, Papastavrou E, et al. The effect of guided imagery on physiological and psychological outcomes of adult ICU patients: A systematic literature review and methodological implications. Aust Crit Care 2018;31(2): 73–86.

Write It Out! CPR for the Soul

Melanie Hall Morris, PhD, APRN, WHNP-BC, CCE

KEYWORDS

• Self-care • Self-compassion • Reflection • Journaling • Well-being

KEY POINTS

- Although expert caregivers for their patients, many nurses routinely neglect to prioritize self-care activities to nurture their own well-being.
- Self-care is not optional for nurses. Lack of self-care can precipitate physical, mental, emotional, spiritual, and social consequences and lead to altered patient outcomes, nurse burnout, and even an exit from the profession.
- Self-compassion can serve as protective shield against burnout while promoting emotional resilience and fostering the ability to compassionately care for others.
- Initiating self-care, or a kind of cardiopulmonary resuscitation for the soul, can mitigate the untoward effects of self-neglect. One option for self-care includes compassionate purposeful reflection or CPR journaling.
- As a cost-effective self-help therapy, CPR journaling applies an "oxygen mask" to help revive and refresh the soul with love, self-compassion, and hope.

INTRODUCTION

With honor comes great responsibility. Being designated by Americans as the most honest and ethical profession for 18 years in a row[1] serves as a wonderful testimony to the influence and the character of the nursing profession. The World Health Organization's (WHO) declaration of 2020 as the Year of the Nurse and the Midwife[2] additionally recognizes nursing's impact. No one could foresee a global pandemic when 2020 was originally deemed the Year of the Nurse and the Midwife, but no one has been surprised by nurses' dedication, commitment, heroism, and sacrifices, including even the loss of life for some nurses, shown during the unprecedented and extremely challenging conditions the pandemic precipitated.

Nurses routinely provide supportive care to patients at all stages of life. Typically, it is nurses who provide the essential care patients receive, whether it be to stimulate and support the initial breaths of a newborn or to hold and comfort patients during their final exhalations. Nurses competently offer the expertise patients can use to navigate

Vanderbilt University School of Nursing, 461 21st Avenue South, Nashville, TN 37240, USA
E-mail address: melanie.h.morris@vanderbilt.edu

Nurs Clin N Am 55 (2020) 475–488
https://doi.org/10.1016/j.cnur.2020.06.014
0029-6465/20/© 2020 Elsevier Inc. All rights reserved.

hurdles created by difficult health-related circumstances. Nurses celebrate with patients the joy of overcoming obstacles and achieving health goals, and nurses do not hesitate to initiate cardiopulmonary resuscitation on any patient whose heart suddenly ceases.

Because of this close care relationship, nurses also find themselves accessible targets for unsatisfied, disgruntled, angry, belligerent, frustrated, and desperate patients who may hurl insults, verbal attacks, and astonishingly even physical punches. It is a reasonable assumption that many nurses chose to enter the nursing profession because of a profound desire to help and care for others during health challenges and likely never considered this decision could possibly impair their own health and well-being.

Although expert caregivers when caring for patients, many nurses routinely tend to overlook extending this expert care to themselves and often struggle to intentionally schedule self-care activities to nurture their own well-being. This neglect can precipitate a myriad of physical, mental, emotional, spiritual, and social consequences that can lead to burnout, or metaphorically a soul arrest, and even an exit from the nursing profession resulting in the "death" of a nursing career.[3,4] Initiating self-care, a kind of cardiopulmonary resuscitation for the soul, offers an antidote for self-care neglect and can perhaps mitigate some of the consequences of this neglect. This article presents a theoretic underpinning for self-care, reasons self-care for nurses is not optional, the benefits of nurses expressing their own stories through journaling, potential barriers associated with journaling, and strategies for implementing cardiopulmonary resuscitation for the soul and using compassionate purposeful reflection (CPR) journaling as a tool to foster well-being.

WATSON'S THEORY OF HUMAN CARING: A SUPPORTIVE FOUNDATION FOR SELF-CARE

Jean Watson[5] writes, "Caring begins with being present, open to compassion, mercy, gentleness, loving-kindness, and equanimity toward and with self before one can offer compassionate caring to others."[5(pxviii)] Watson's 10 Caritas Processes, which evolved from 10 Carative Factors, function as a basis for professional nurses to apply the caring theory's constructs in their practices.[5,6] The first Caritas Process, "sustaining humanistic-altruistic values by practice of lovingkindness, compassion, and equanimity with self/others,"[6(p22)] offers a plausible foundation for self-care. In addition, this first Caritas Process proposes that to authentically care for others, self-care and self-compassion in the caregiver are vital.[6]

Nurses endeavor to provide beneficent care to all patients. However, nurses may find it difficult to give the same loving-kindness to themselves that they extend effortlessly to others.[6] The ancient text of The Bible declares in Matthew 22:39, "You shall love your neighbor as [you do] yourself" (The Amplified Bible). Loving and caring for oneself makes it possible to provide care to others. Not properly caring for oneself can affect one's capacity to care but also affects the quality of the care given.[7]

Using Watson's[5] theory of caring, Hernandez[8] suggested a self-care model for nurses based on the acronym CARING: C for self-compassion, A for awareness, R for reflection, I for intentionality, N for nonjudgmental attachment, and G for gratitude.[8] Incorporating these concepts offers a practical approach to self-care. Watson[5] suggested meditation, mindfulness, self-awareness, journaling, prayer, using positive affirmations, enjoying nature, practicing gratitude, forgiveness, and silence as concrete ways to implement the first Caritas Process of sustaining loving-kindness to self and others.[5] In addition, practical application of this process includes consistently practicing loving-kindness with oneself, no matter the circumstances.[6]

SELF-CARE IS NOT OPTIONAL FOR NURSES

More than ever, during the recent global pandemic the sentiment that nurses are heroes has resonated in many places. However, all heroes, regardless of the "super-powers" they may possess, must pause long enough to refuel their "soul tanks" and recharge their batteries through personal self-care, so they can continue to offer their best selves as they care for their patients. Self-care includes attention to physical needs such as adequate sleep, healthy nutrition, and fitness as well as care of mental, emotional, and spiritual needs through stress management techniques, hobby pursuits, and spiritual practices.[7] However, within a profession founded on providing care for others, many nurses routinely neglect to prioritize self-care even to the extent of postponing basic self-care needs, such as eating and toileting, during a hectic work shift.

Remnants from the emotional investment of caring for patients can linger long after the workday ends for nurses. No control button exists to turn off caring and stop the continued thoughts related to the patients. A key finding from the American Nurses Association (ANA) Health Risk Appraisal revealed that 68% of 10,688 nurses surveyed indicated that they put the well-being (health, safety, and wellness) of their patients before their own.[9] A qualitative study of health care professionals, mostly nurses and student nurses, echoed similar results.[10] These findings, although not shocking, cause concern, especially given that the ANA deems self-care important enough to include it as 1 of the 9 provisions in the Code of Ethics for Nurses.[11] Just as vehicles cannot operate without proper fuel or electricity, nurses cannot expect to function effectively when their self-care needs go unmet. Therefore, when considering how to balance caring for patients with personal well-being, nurses must make routine self-care interventions a priority.

Respecting oneself naturally incorporates love and care for self, providing a strong foundation for giving enlightened care to others.[12] Caring for self first makes it possible to care for others, and, in order to gain or retain the energy required to compassionately care for others, this care of self is essential.[13] Extending intentional care to others can transform the surrounding environment, reaching well beyond the initial recipient much like a ripple through a tranquil pond caused by 1 dropped pebble.[12]

Orem's self-care theory, as cited by McKirvergin and colleagues,[14(p79)] defines self-care as "the practice of activities that individuals initiate and perform on their own behalf in maintaining life, health, and well-being." Self-care, a necessity for self-preservation, is far from selfish and not optional for nurses. Practicing self-care contributes to wellness, promotes resilience, and improves passion for life while helping to buffer against stress and frustration,[15] thus serving a critical role in promoting healing at the cellular level, protecting against disease triggers,[4] and creating calm within the mind, body, and spirit. Nurses' self-assessment, self-reflection, and self-care promotes personal growth and development, contributing to their well-being and equipping them for service to others.[16]

A holistic approach to self-care includes attending to all dimensions of one's being. These aspects of self as described by Dossey and Keegan[17] include the components physical, mental, emotions, relationships, choices, and spirit that together comprise the wholeness of human potentials. Continually interacting, all dimensions are significant and required to perpetuate wholeness.[17]

Each of us has the ability to achieve a balanced integration of human potentials: physical, mental, emotions, relationships, choices, and spirit. Effective self-care and self-healing depend on taking all of these potentials into account. We are challenged to gain access to our inner wisdom and intuition and apply them in our daily lives. As we take responsibility for making effective choices and changes in our lives, we place ourselves in a better position to clarify our life patterns, purposes, and processes.[18(p377)]

A key component of self-care includes learning to quieten or to soothe one's own emotional or physical distress.[19] Self-care activities are purposeful, and self-care does not encompass self-indulgence behaviors such as television bingeing for hours while consuming unhealthy snacks.[19] Although it might be tempting to justify or rationalize so-called vegging-out activities as earned or deserved, these behaviors can sabotage other more beneficial self-care efforts and subsequently increase the body's stress response even more.[19]

Pampering oneself with self-care treats, such as manicures, pedicures, or a shopping spree, may bring temporary relief from distress and feel like optimal self-care, but making the effort to incorporate health-seeking self-care behaviors best mitigates life's stressors.[19] Self-care activities such as adequate sleep; healthy nutrition; consistent exercise; and using stress reduction tactics such as meditation, mindfulness, journaling, relaxation, or yoga aid in balancing work and home responsibilities.[4,5,12,19]

Consequences of Self-Care Neglect

An inattention to self can create a self-care deficit. If this self-negligence continues, it can trigger physical and mental symptoms such as obesity, hypertension, anxiety, depression, fatigue, insomnia, and/or immune system dysfunction, any of which can contribute to compassion fatigue, burnout, and even nurses leaving the profession.[3,4]

Nurses' perpetual giving of self both emotionally and physically to patients' care without providing loving-kindness to the self can take its toll[5] and leave the nurse feeling empty. An imbalance in any facet of life often produces a ripple effect, disturbing the equilibrium and the level of functioning.[12] This ripple effect can continue to extend beyond the nurse and begin to affect outcomes in patients on the receiving end of care. Mental, physical, and emotional exhaustion interfere with observational skills and performance. Intense stress hinders the ability to use higher-level thinking skills, forcing nurses into a survival mode, a lower functioning level of the brain.[20] Although unintentional, when nurses function at less than their best because of burnout, the opportunities increase for subtle patient condition changes to be missed or ignored, consequently compromising patient safety as well as patient outcomes.[7,21]

SELF-COMPASSION

Self-compassion is described as treating oneself with the same kindness and thoughtfulness given to any friend.[22,23] Self-compassion extends kindness, understanding, and mercy to oneself, countering the negative self-accusations, self-blame, and self-criticism when faced with perceived inadequacies or failures.[24] Self-compassion also can boost a positive mindset.[24]

What does self-compassion look like? It "means becoming your own best friend."[23(p21)] Who can be a better friend than one's own self? No one knows you any better than your own self does. Nurses must realize they are worthy of the same nurturing and compassion[25] they shower on their patients. Furthermore, most nurses would never utter disparaging words to patients, associates, or even strangers regardless of the circumstances. However, nurses often become their own worst critics, speaking unkind and harsh words to themselves using both their inner and external audible voices whenever they fail to meet their own expectations.[26]

For people who find self-compassion challenging, developing the practice is feasible[22] and is often associated with practicing mindfulness.[27] Self-criticism declines with the increase of self-compassion, and this can inspire more achievement and giving of self.[22] Self-criticism may be associated with the fight-or-flight response, increasing stress hormone levels in the body, whereas self-compassion may signal the physiologic release of oxytocin, the hormone of attachment and love.[22]

Self-compassion can foster the ability to continue to care for others while serving as a protective shield against decreased resilience and caregiver burnout.[27,28] Self-compassion can promote emotional resilience and psychological well-being.[24,29,30]

POSITIVE PSYCHOLOGY

Martin Seligman, a pioneer in positive psychology, inaugurated the new field in 1998.[31] Applied positive psychology, the label for "the science and practice of improving well-being,"[31(p1347)] uses practical interventions to facilitate well-being.[31] Substituting negative thoughts with positive perspectives and actions stimulates the centers in the brain responsible for creation, production, motivation, and resilience.[32] Positivity can trigger a release of the so-called feel-good hormones, dopamine and serotonin; decrease the body's inflammatory reaction caused by stress; boost the performance of the immune system; and alter the brain's structure.[33]

Mindfulness meditation can help to refocus the mind and can vitally contribute to positive well-being by expanding the happiness in the brain.[32] Possessing high subjective well-being could potentially add 4 to 10 years of more enjoyable life compared with perceptions of low subjective well-being.[34] Gratitude journaling serves as an example of a practical positive psychology intervention.[31]

NEUROPLASTICITY

Neuroplasticity describes the dynamic capability of the brain to continuously adapt and change.[35] This ability of the brain to change its structure and function creates the capacity for the mind to heal.[7] One's experiences as well as mental activity such as one's thoughts and emotions can trigger these brain changes, which can affect the body.[36,37]

Self-directed neuroplasticity refers to the capacity to direct alterations in the brain through focused attention in a positive or negative direction.[38] Cultivating an attitude of gratitude develops different brain circuitry than when one's attention repeatedly focuses on a list of complaints.[38] Changing one's thinking can be life changing. By shifting thinking to a more positive perspective, the brain creatively redirects the neural pathways toward these more prevalent thoughts, beliefs, and emotions.[38]

Writing can affect the neuroplasticity of the brain, facilitating the brain's ability to purposefully transform in healthy ways.[38] Any type of journaling compels people to pause, ponder, and put in writing specific thoughts and ideas, and in essence creates a tangible way to encourage mindfulness in the moment. Journaling offers a way for nurses to emotionally support and sustain themselves in their work efforts.[39]

EXPRESSING YOUR STORY WITH JOURNALING
Reflection

Jack Mezirow[40] fittingly describes reflection in the following way.

*Reflection, a 'turning back' on experience, can mean many things: simple aware-
ness of an object, event or state, including awareness of a perception, thought,
feeling, disposition, intention, action, or of one's habits of doing these things. It
can also mean letting one's thoughts wander over something, taking something
into consideration, or imaging alternatives. One can reflect on oneself
reflecting.[40(p185)]*

The nature of the work nurses perform inevitably leads to frequent reflection. Mulling
over planned actions, present actions, or past actions occurs throughout every
workday regardless of whether these actions are recognized as reflection. Nurses
use reflection automatically following unexpected events or the occurrence of unanticipated patient outcomes. This reflection on the care provided is essential and contributes to the development and refinement of expert practice skills.[41] Reflection is
integrated within all of the steps of the nursing process and is considered to be a significant process in the development of nurses who are capable and compassionate.[41]
Self-reflection can serve as a useful coping strategy for gaining an accurate perspective of situations.[42]

Daniel Pesut, former President of the Honor Society of Nursing, Sigma Theta Tau
International, shared the following thoughts about the essence and purpose of reflection in nursing in reference to the society's newly created resource article on the scholarship of reflection.

*Personally and professionally I believe reflection is a means of renewal. My logic
goes something like this: as self is renewed, commitments to service come forward more easily. Renewed commitments to service require attention to mindfulness and reflective practice. Mindful reflective practice begets questions that
support inquiry. Such inquiry guides knowledge work and evidence-based care
giving. Care giving supports society as knowledge, values, and service intersect.
Knowledgeable people and especially knowledgeable nurses provide care that
society needs. Creating a caring society is the spirit work of nursing. Creating a
caring society starts nurses caring for themselves and becoming, through reflection, more conscious and intentional in their being, thinking, feeling, doing, and
acting. Reflection is a form of "inner work" that results in the energy for engaging
in "outer service." Reflection in-and-on action supports meaning-making and purpose management in one's professional life.[39(p1)]*

Reflection involves the sharing of one's story. Most people enjoy hearing or reading
a good story. A good story commands attention. A good story enthralls and mesmer-
izes. A well-told story can evoke a range of sentiments prompting outward expressions of emotions such as tears and laughter. Good stories can stimulate creativity.
Sharing a story can validate an experience while providing an opportunity to build connections between people, places, and ideas. However, opportunities for growth are
overlooked when storytelling ends with verbal expression only.

Journaling: Sharing a Story

Journaling offers a means to apply the process of reflection[7,41] and provides an excellent foundation for reflective thinking.[43] Journaling presents the opportunity to tell a
story: your own. Without judgment, censorship, or editorial corrections, journaling allows the freedom to write it out from the perspective of the person who knows the
story best: you. The mere act of writing one's story promotes self-reflection and can
serve as a source of revelation, encouragement, rejuvenation, and even healing, in
essence like cardiopulmonary resuscitation for the soul. Loehr[44] declares that an
intentional rewiring of the brain can result from writing one's story in long hand and

can serve as one of the most powerful ways to change one's story. "Self-reflection is a special kind of nurturing that enhances our soul and its expression,"[45(p47)] and release of emotions through journaling can improve health and well-being.[43]

Benefits of Journaling

Carving out time to continue to express one's story by writing through journaling may offer powerful benefits. Hiemstra[46] describes journaling as an "investment in self through a growing awareness of personal thoughts and feelings."[46(p24)] Not only can journaling promote personal growth, it provides an opportunity for reflection, critical thinking, and problem solving.[46] Listening to one's inner voice and writing one's thoughts through journaling can help reduce stress and improve health.[46] Journaling offers a way to care for oneself while also enhancing the awareness and concern with caring for others.[25]

Expressive writing through journaling restores balance and peace and initiates change within.[38] Expressive writing can potentially "change the way you see the world."[47(pxiv)] Writing can function as a bridge connecting one to aspects of self that have been uncared for and disregarded, the aspects of self that possess wisdom and want the best for ourselves.[38] Writing can help to rediscover the inner voice of kindheartedness that tends to get silenced by the berating and chastising messages sent by the typically louder inner critical voice.

Pausing to journal creates space to think and listen to one's kind inner voice, much like communicating with a best friend, and perhaps can trigger a change in one's perspective of a situation. Being attuned to the private, inner voice that no one else hears, the master storyteller that possesses powerful influence over one's future trajectory, aids in getting one's own story accurate, which then can contribute to clarity in moving forward.[48] Learning to use the powerful inner voices of support, encouragement, and compassion may require practice and repetition, much like weightlifting helps to strengthen muscles.[48]

Journaling can be transformational. It is self-help therapy that assists with life management and can lead to physical and emotional healing as well as the prevention of burnout.[49] A journal truly is "your companion, your therapist, your best friend, your teacher, your punching bag, and your personal historian all rolled up in a simple book. It's inexpensive and easy to use – and it doesn't talk back."[50(p4)] The journaling process lends itself to dialogue, whether it be with oneself, someone else, or someone in one's imagination.[46]

Journaling also allows for the dumping of nonbeneficial thoughts from the mind that serve no purpose and take up space. Freeing the mind of these thoughts opens up more room for creativity, problem solving, and positivity. Writing it out acts as a powerful tool for supporting mindfulness, facilitating self-compassion, and allowing the expression of emotions promoting health and well-being.[43] Recording thoughts gives them a place to dwell outside of the mind and can function as a symbolic letting go of the power and negativity associated with them. In addition, by tearing up, throwing away, or burning the written evidence, one may even experience a new sense of release and freedom. Journaling offers such a cost-effective approach to self-therapy, including the immense benefit of round-the-clock availability, that it might be hard to imagine it can be effective.

In a study with 66 registered nurses who participated in a 6-week program comprising six 2.5-hour journaling classes, journaling was found to decrease burnout and compassion fatigue while increasing compassion satisfaction.[51] Participants indicated that journaling served as an outlet for expressing thoughts and feelings therapeutically, assisted them in decision-making on the job, and facilitated the ability to take care of themselves, which in turn helped them better care for others.[51]

Fifteen Registered Nurse (RN) to Bachelor of Science students reported that reflective journaling prompted engagement in self-care and health promotion practices by reducing stress and bringing clarity to thoughts.[52] Implementing a 6-week positive writing intervention showed a statistically significant increased level of optimism and gratitude in mothers of troubled children.[53] In this same mixed-methods study, positive thinking, emotional well-being, and mental health self-care emerged as the major themes.[53] The journaling exercise increased awareness of gratitude, provided relaxation, and was an effective stress management tool.[53]

Physical and psychological benefits noted from journaling include decreased blood pressure and depressive symptoms and improved emotional regulation, cognition, insight, and immune functioning.[43,54,55] Although benefits continue to be noted through research as well as anecdotally, journaling for reflection and self-care continues to be an overlooked practical option.[43]

Barriers that Interfere with Journaling

Time constraints and obligations related to responsibilities from multiple caregiving roles associated with work, family, and others can interfere with establishing and maintaining journaling practices. Common barriers for journaling include perceived lack of time and calendars filled with commitments making it challenging to prioritize a journaling activity.[53] Lack of confidence in ability to write can also present an obstacle.[56]

Choosing to overlook journaling as a viable option for self-care before even trying it can deprive one of many of the potential benefits already outlined. Hesitation because of perceived barriers can be addressed with specific strategies and should not prevent one from jumping in and determining a journaling practice that can work. Recommendations and strategies for overcoming common barriers associated with journaling are listed in **Table 1**.

Cardiopulmonary Resuscitation for the Soul: Compassionate Purposeful Reflection (CPR) Journaling

For patients with cardiac arrest, prompt cardiopulmonary resuscitation maintains perfusion of the patient's vital organs, which significantly increases the patient's chance for survival.[57] In the same way that nurses initiate cardiopulmonary resuscitation when a patient's heartbeat ceases to perfuse the body effectively with life-sustaining oxygen, nurses should consider implementing a kind of cardiopulmonary resuscitation for the soul to perfuse their bodies with self-care life support. Cardiopulmonary resuscitation for the soul can help to mitigate the sequelae of compassion fatigue and burnout or soul arrest and perhaps increase the long-term survival of a nursing career. With prompt attention and a focus on their own individual self-care needs, nurses can discover and participate in activities that consistently refuel and recharge their soul tanks. Full soul tanks increase nurses' capability to function effectively and care compassionately.

Cardiopulmonary resuscitation for the soul can be implemented in a variety of ways and will differ between nurses. One option for filling one's soul tank includes compassionate purposeful reflection or CPR journaling. Benefits have been noted when time is spent to hand write reflective thoughts, and this offers a way to apply a needed oxygen mask, helping to revive and refresh the soul with love, self-compassion, and hope. CPR journaling can aid in replenishing depleted stores of resilience and compassion.

Table 1
Common journaling barriers and strategies to overcome

Barrier	Potential Strategy to Overcome Barrier
Not knowing where to begin	Starting with a blank page or a journal can be overwhelming. Many people are not sure where to begin. Remember, there is no right or wrong. This is for you. If you need a little help in starting, review this Web page. https://www.rachaelkable.com/blog/how-to-use-a-blank-journal
Not having enough time	In a busy profession this is a reality, but there are ways to work through this. For example, start with bullet points rather than full sentences. Journal weekly or biweekly instead of daily. Start the journal with specifics. For example, name 3 positive things that occurred recently or 3 things for which you are thankful. Use a convenient time to journal regularly, such as coffee breaks, before going to bed, or during television commercials. Journal for a set amount of time (eg, 5, 7, or 10 min) and then stop
Having a tough day	Having a tough day may make people think that journaling is the last thing they want to do today. However, journaling may boost your mood as discussed and support your well-being. Start with thoughts such as, "I smiled today because......" or "Today, I am really glad that I...." Identify a positive experience then elaborate in the journal
Lack of motivation	When tired, it is easy to procrastinate with nonessential tasks. Think of rewarding yourself for journaling. Promise yourself a favorite beverage, snack, television program, or any other interest you enjoy after journaling
Misplacing your journaling tools	Keep your journal and a writing tool in the same place so they are conveniently accessible when you are ready to journal. Taking time to find your journal or writing tool can diminish your enthusiasm and become frustrating
Feeling you are bad at journaling	There are often ebbs and flows with journaling. Remember, this is just for you. Journaling is part of a journey and not a destination. If you experience a slump, set it aside for a while. Come back to it when you are ready or perhaps even try a different method. For example, use a gratitude approach or write a letter to a friend. The right or perfect way to journal is the way that fits best for you

Adapted from: Kabel R. Ten obstacles that stop you from journaling and how to overcome them! https://www.rachaelkable.com/blog/journaling-obstacles Accessed May 21, 2020.

STRATEGIES FOR IMPLEMENTING CARDIOPULMONARY RESUSCITATION FOR THE SOUL
Self-Care Contracts

As part of curriculum requirements, RN students in a Bachelor of Science in Nursing degree program created self-care contracts during each semester that identified specific activities they planned to implement to promote self-care.[58] These nurses acknowledged the value of self-care contracts, indicating that the contracts gave them official permission to take time to enjoy activities without feeling guilty, and they also noted positive benefits of decreased stress and improved wellness of body, mind, and spirit.[58]

Self-care activities, including designating time for exercise, eating properly, sleeping, and socializing with friends, should be added and scheduled into a weekly calendar.[59] Adding a separate me-time meeting on one's calendar identifies dedicated time for pursuing activities with self or others that will refresh and rejuvenate. Intentionally committing to this scheduled time and avoiding the temptation to cancel or reschedule reinforces the value self-care.

Ideas for Implementing Journaling

Commonly, when one considers journaling, writing words about daily events and/or associated emotions comes to mind. However, any type of written expression in the form of poems, songs, sketches, drawings, doodles, and stream-of-consciousness writings can be added to journals.[60] In addition, color and images can be integrated in this self-expression, producing a unique depiction of one's way of experiencing.[60]

Kathleen Adams, a pioneer in journal therapy and the founder/director of the Center for Journal Therapy and the Therapeutic Writing Institute based in Colorado, offers reports, books, conferences, retreats, online courses, and a variety of free resources through her Web site[61] as well as tips for getting started at https://journaltherapy.com/lets-journal/a-short-course-in-journal-writing/. Adams[62] created a model called the Journal Ladder with 14 writing techniques from her Journal Toolbox. The lower rungs of the Journal Ladder include more concrete, structured, and paced journal therapy activities that are more informational in nature, such as sentence completion prompts, short timed focused writing, and a quick assessment of various aspects of one's life.[62] Moving up the ladder, the writing techniques progress to increasingly more insightful, intuitive, and abstract activities with less structure, such as writing from an alternate perspective, writing as if metaphorically conversing with another, and writing with no imposed boundaries.[62]

To begin journaling, just start. Write even if it is only a few words or for only a limited amount of time. Participants learning journaling techniques indicated surprise that, in as few as 5 minutes of writing, they noted increased clarity, generation of new ideas, and potential options for problems that had been previously overlooked.[62] The following prompt, WRITE, adapted from Ross and Adams,[38] can serve as a guide:

W: write. Determine what you want to write about and just write (Prompt suggestions: What am I thinking? How am I feeling?).
R: reconnect by taking a few moments to breathe deeply, relax, and center yourself.
I: investigate. Consider your thoughts and feelings and then write without editing.
T: time it. Set a timer and write for a particular amount of time, reserving the final few minutes for reflection and wrap-up.
E: exit purposefully; review and reflect. Wrap up with 1 or 2 sentences about what you noticed or thought. Jot down any next actions and ideas for a subsequent writing session.[38]

Another idea is to generate a simple joy list. Creating a joy list challenges nurses to focus on things loved and, therefore, may precipitate ideas that can be incorporated into self-care activities.[63] Think about any interests or activities that bring peace, joy, and contentment. As this list of options grows, prioritize each endeavor. Just as nursing care includes assessing, planning, and implementing a care plan for each patient, take the time to devise an individualized self-care plan to inspire, refresh, and stimulate joy. Plan the specific details of how to implement an option from the list and then just do it.

Consider starting with a gratitude list. "Gratitude is open-heart therapy."[8(p132)] Actively practicing gratitude can foster contentment and happiness within oneself

Box 1
Suggestions for developing a journaling habit
1. Be real: strive to be authentic. Avoid the urge to censor your writing.
2. Protect your privacy: vital for facilitating honesty when writing.
3. Handwrite your thoughts: encourages the development and connections of thoughts.
4. Create a dedicated space for quiet reflection without distractions.
5. Determine a convenient time, schedule an appointment with yourself, and show up: begin slowly (weekly, biweekly, or monthly) and increase frequency, aiming for a daily designated time.
6. Include the date (and time) of each entry. Allows the opportunity to note changes and growth.
7. Give yourself permission to pause when you need a temporary hiatus.
8. Keep it simple when establishing routines, creating expectations, and choosing tools and words to use.
Data from Scott SJ, Davenport B. *Effortless Journaling: How to Start a Journal, Make it a Habit, and Find Endless Writing Topics,* "8 Rules for Consistent Journaling." Cranbury, NJ: Oldtown Publishing LLC; 2018, pp. 123-129.

that is not influenced by external situations.[8] Developing gratitude through journaling has been noted to decrease stress and contribute to improved well-being.[64] Conducting a quick Internet search using the keywords "gratitude journal prompts" can yield many associated blogs with tips providing a free and easy way to get started.

Box 1 includes several ideas for creating a consistent journaling habit. Incorporate 1 or all of the suggestions to begin a simple journaling routine.

SUMMARY

Self-care is essential for nurses, whose work is the business of caring for others. Cultivating time for thoughtful and compassionate reflective journaling can result in a variety of physical, mental, emotional, and spiritual benefits. CPR journaling can be a life-sustaining and effective self-care tool for nurses, especially when caregiving for others has drained their joy and resilience stores, leaving them feeling depleted. The key is to create time and space, even if it is only 5 minutes, for reflection filled with self-compassion. Try it. It is almost a guarantee that this dedicated space of time for self-care through CPR journaling will become a desired activity and something to look forward to doing. Make concrete plans to battle any barriers and implement the journaling strategies that resonate in whatever manner works optimally. Regardless of the method used, frequency of occurrence, or length of time spent, regularly pursue occasions to implement CPR journaling for the soul and just write it out!

REFERENCES

1. Brusie C. Nurses Ranked Most Honest Profession 18 Years in a Row. nurse.org. 2020. Available at: https://nurse.org/articles/nursing-ranked-most-honest-profession/. Accessed April 29, 2020.
2. Year of the Nurse and the Midwife 2020. World Health Organization; 2020. Available at: https://www.who.int/news-room/campaigns/year-of-the-nurse-and-the-midwife-2020. Accessed April 29, 2020.

3. Kravits K, McAllister-Black R, Grant M, et al. Self-care strategies for nurses: A psycho-educational intervention for stress reduction and the prevention of burnout. Appl Nurs Res 2010;23(3):130–8.

4. Richards K. Wellpower: The foundation of innovation. Nurs Econ 2013;31(2):94–8.

5. Watson J. Nursing: the philosophy and science of caring. Revised edition. Boulder (CO): University Press of Colorado; 2008. Available at: www.jstor.org/stable/j.ctt1d8h9wn.

6. Sitzman K, Watson J. Caring science, mindful practice: implementing Watson's human caring theory. 2nd edition. New York: Springer Publishing Company, LLC; 2018.

7. Kreitzer MJ. Integrative nursing: Application of principles across clinical settings. Rambam Maimonides Med J 2015;6(2). https://doi.org/10.5041/RMMJ.10200.

8. Hernandez G. The heART of self-C.A.R.I.N.G.: A journey to becoming an optimal healing presence to ourselves and our patients. Creat Nurs 2009;15(3):129–33.

9. Executive summary: American nurses association health Risk appraisal (key findings: October 2013-October 2016). 2017. Available at: https://www.nursingworld.org/~495c56/globalassets/practiceandpolicy/healthy-nurse-healthy-nation/ana-healthriskappraisalsummary_2013-2016.pdf. Accessed May 4, 2020.

10. Egan H, Keyte R, McGowan K, et al. 'You before me': A qualitative study of health care professionals' and students' understanding and experiences of compassion in the workplace, self-compassion, self-care and health behaviours. Health Professions Education 2019;5(3):225–36.

11. American Nurses Association. Code of Ethics for Nurses with Interpretive Statements. 2015. Available at: https://www.nursingworld.org/practice-policy/nursing-excellence/ethics/code-of-ethics-for-nurses/. Accessed May 4, 2020.

12. Sitzman KL. Teaching-learning professional caring based on Jean Watson's Theory of Human Caring. Int J Hum Caring 2007;11(4):8–16.

13. Turkel MC, Ray MA. Creating a caring practice environment through self-renewal. Nurs Adm Q 2004;28(4):249–54.

14. McKivergin M, Wimberly T, Loversidge J, et al. Creating a work environment that supports self-care. Holist Nurs Pract 1996;10(2):78–88.

15. Uno K, Ruthman JL. Wellness as a self-care philosophy for nurses and their leaders. Holist Nurs Pract 2006;20(1):3–4.

16. Mariano C. Holistic nursing as a specialty: Holistic nursing—scope and standards of practice. Nurs Clin North Am 2007;42(2):165–88.

17. Dossey BM, Keegan L. Self-assessments: facilitating healing in self and others. In: Dossey BM, Keegan L, Guzzetta CE, editors. Holistic nursing: a handbook for practice. 4th edition. Sudbury (MA): Jones & Bartlett Learning; 2005. p. 379–93.

18. Dossey BM, Keegan L, Guzzetta CE. Holistic nursing: a handbook for practice. 4th edition. Sudbury (MA): Jones & Bartlett Learning; 2005. Available at: http://proxy.library.vanderbilt.edu/login?url=http://search.ebscohost.com/login.aspx?direct=true&db=nlebk&AN=128408&site=ehost-live&scope=site. Accessed May, 19, 2020.

19. Richards K. Self-care is a lifelong journey. Nurs Econ 2013;31(4):198–202.

20. Holmes K. Neuroscience, mindfulness and holistic wellness reflections on interconnectivity in teaching and learning. Interchange 2019;50(3):445–60.

21. Spence Laschinger HK, Leiter M. The impact of nursing work environments on patient safety outcomes: The mediating role of burnout engagement. J Nurs Adm 2006;36(5):259–67.

22. Seppala E. Self-Compassion. Spirituality & Health Magazine 2011. Available at: https://link.gale.com/apps/doc/A270373853/AONE?u=tel_a_vanderbilt&sid=AONE&xid=5d68e249. Accessed May 1, 2020.

23. Sheridan C. The mindful nurse: using the power of mindfulness and compassion to help you thrive in your work. Rivertime Press; 2016. Available at: www.rivertimepress.com.

24. Warren R, Smeets E, Neff K. Self-criticism and self-compassion: Risk and resilience: Being compassionate to oneself is associated with emotional resilience and psychological well-being. Curr Psychiatr 2016;15(12):18–21, 24-28, 32.

25. Charles JP. Journaling: creating space for "I. Creat Nurs 2010;16(4):180–4.

26. McKee A, Wiens K. Prevent burnout by making compassion a habit. Harv Business Rev 2017. Available at: https://hbr.org/2017/05/prevent-burnout-by-making-compassion-a-habit. Accessed April 29, 2020.

27. Neff K. The 5 myths of self-compassion: What keeps us from being kinder to ourselves? Psychotherapy Networker 2015;39(5). Available at: https://search-proquest-com.proxy.library.vanderbilt.edu/docview/1721325775?rfr_id=info%3Axri%2Fsid%3Aprimo. Accessed May 2, 2020.

28. Coaston SC. Self-care through self-compassion: A balm for burnout. The Professional Counselor 2017;7(3):285–97.

29. Germer CK, Neff KD. Self-compassion in clinical practice. J Clin Psychol 2013; 69(8):856–67.

30. Neff KD, Kirkpatrick KL, Rude SS. Self-compassion and adaptive psychological functioning. J Res Pers 2007;41(1):139–54.

31. Lomas T, Hefferon K, Ivtzan I. The LIFE Model: A meta-theoretical conceptual map for applied positive psychology. J Happiness Stud 2015;16(5):1347–64.

32. Walker D. The meaning of happiness: Strategies for pursuing and obtaining happiness. Am Nurse Today 2018;13(4):30.

33. Fredrickson B. Positivity. Crown Publishers; 2009.

34. Diener E, Chan MY. Happy people live longer: Subjective well-being contributes to health and longevity. Appl Psychol Health Well Being 2011;3(1):1–43.

35. Choy L. Neuroplasticity and mental wellness: Our path forward. In: Bodeker G, editor. Mental wellness white paper. Global Wellness Institute; 2017. p. 18–29.

36. Davidson RJ. The neurobiology of compassion. In: Germer CK, Siegel RD, editors. Wisdom and compassion in psychotherapy: deepening mindfulness in clinical practice. New York: Guilford Press; 2012. p. 111–8.

37. Quinn K. Something is going to happen here: The use of mandala art in enhancing reflective practice. ANS Adv Nurs Sci 2019;42(3):E1–19.

38. Ross D, Adams K. Your brain on ink: a workbook on neuroplasticity and the journal ladder. Workbook edition. Lanham (MD): Rowman & Littlefield; 2016.

39. Sherwood G, Freshwater D, Horton-Deutsch S, et al. Sigma Theta Tau International's resource paper on the Scholarship of reflective practice. The Honor Society of Nursing, Sigma Theta Tau International; 2005. p. 31. Available at: https://www.sigmanursing.org/docs/default-source/position-papers/resource_reflective.pdf?sfvrsn=4.

40. Mezirow J. On critical reflection. Adult Educ Q 1998;48(3):185–98.

41. Lauterbach SS, Hentz PB. Journaling to learn: A strategy in nursing education for developing the nurse as a person and person as nurse. Int J Hum Caring 2005; 9(1):29–35.

42. Upton KV. An investigation into compassion fatigue and self-compassion in acute medical care hospital nurses: A mixed methods study. Journal of Compassionate Healthcare 2018;5(7):1–27.

43. Dimitroff LJ. Journaling: A valuable tool for registered nurses. Am Nurse Today 2018;13(11):27–8.
44. Jim Loehr. The power of story 2017. Available at: https://www.youtube.com/watch?v=D_0NnqkmVM4. Accessed May 17, 2020.
45. Drick CA. Nurturing yourself to enhance your practice. Int J Childbirth Educ 2014; 29(1):46–51.
46. Hiemstra R. Uses and benefits of journal writing. New Dir Adult Cont Educ 2001;(90):19–26.
47. Adams K. Expressive writing: foundations of Practice. Lanham (MD): Rowman & Littlefield Education; 2013.
48. Loehr J. The power of story: rewrite your destiny in business and in life. New York: Free Press; 2007.
49. McCarthy ML. Journaling power: how to create the happy, healthy life you want to live. Hasmark Publishing; 2016.
50. Scott SJ, Davenport B. Effortless journaling: how to start a journal, make a habit, and find endless writing. Oldtown Publishing LLC; 2018.
51. Dimitroff LJ, Sliwoski L, O'Brien S, et al. Change your life through journaling–The benefits of journaling for registered nurses. J Nurs Educ Pract 2017;7(2):90–8.
52. Padykula BM. RN-BS students' reports of their self-care and health promotion practices in a holistic nursing course. J Holist Nurs 2017;35(3):221–46.
53. Kim-Godwin YS, Kim S-S, Gil M. Journaling for self-care and coping in mothers of troubled children in the community. Arch Psychiatr Nurs 2020;34(2):50–7.
54. Baikie KA, Wilhelm K. Emotional and physical health benefits of expressive writing. Adv Psychiatr Treat 2005;11(5):338–46.
55. Sexton JD, Pennebaker JW, Holzmueller CG, et al. Care for the caregiver: Benefits of expressive writing for nurses in the United States. Prog Palliat Care 2009; 17(6):307–12.
56. Hayman B, Wikes L, Jackson D. Journaling: Identification of challenges and reflection on strategies. Nurse Res 2012;19(3):27–31.
57. American Heart Association. What is CPR? CPR & First Aid: Emergency Cardiovascular Care. 2020. Available at: https://cpr.heart.org/en/resources/what-is-cpr. Accessed May 1, 2020.
58. Ellis LL. Have you and your staff signed self-care contracts? Nurs Manag 2000; 31(3):47–78.
59. Cline C, Frolic A, Sibbald R. Beyond trail blazing: A roadmap for new healthcare ethics leaders (and the people who hire them). HEC Forum 2013;25(3):211–27.
60. Boud D. Using journal writing to enhance reflective practice. New Dir Adult Cont Educ 2001;2001(90):9–17.
61. Adams K. The center for journal therapy. Wheat Ridge (CO): The Center for Journal Therapy; 2018. Available at: https://journaltherapy.com/. Accessed May 19, 2020.
62. Adams K. The journal ladder: a developmental continuum of journal therapy. 2011. Available at: https://journaltherapy.com/wp-content/uploads/2011/01/CJT_Journal_Ladder-FINAL.pdf. Accessed May 19, 2020.
63. Krischke MM. Nurse leaders offer wisdom on achieving work-life balance. NurseZone Newsletter 2011.
64. Emmons RA, Froh J, Rose R. Gratitude. In: Gallagher MW, Lopez SJ, editors. Positive psychological assessment: a handbook of models and measures. 2nd edition. Washington, DC: Publications and Reports of the Surgeon General. American Psychological Association; 2019. p. 317–32. https://doi.org/10.1037/0000138-020.

Clinical Aromatherapy

Ashley J. Farrar, BSN, RN[a], Francisca C. Farrar, EdD, MSN, RN[b],*

KEYWORDS

- Clinical aromatherapy • Clinical management • Best practice model • History
- Theoretic frameworks • Plant sources • Safety case reports • Pathologic response

KEY POINTS

- Aromatherapy is an alternative medicine or integrative therapy that works with conventional medicine treatment.
- The Food and Drug Administration of the United States guidelines classify essential oils as cosmetics because they are not drugs for treating or prevention of disease.
- Essential oils come from seeds, stems, leaves, needles, petals, flowers, rinds and fruits, woods and resins, roots and rhizomes, and grasses.
- Case reports are presented for considerations regarding flammability, elder and child safety, dermatitis, phototoxicity, oral toxicity, and eye safety, including critical analysis and intervention.
- Clinical aromatherapy can be beneficial for symptom management for pain, nausea, vomiting, preoperative anxiety, critical care, well-being, anxiety, depression, stress, insomnia, respiratory, dementia, and oncology.

INTRODUCTION

The Western perspective on health care has been focused on medications for treatment of health care conditions. It was common for pain to be treated with various levels of opioids and receiving prescriptions for medications with each physician visit. Sadly, over time, opioids and antianxiety medications were abused, with the result of these medications purchased from drug dealers, overdosing, and death. The federal government and states stepped in, passing laws monitoring prescriptions written for opioids; therefore, a search for alternative medicine began. Alternative methods were found in the Eastern perspective on health care. Yoga, Pilates, mindfulness meditation, acupuncture, and scented oils were used with massage. Westerners found many alternative methods to treat medical conditions, such as pain, anxiety, depression, and insomnia, with scented oils from various plant sources. The pendulum began to swing from Western medication to an Eastern holistic approach. Aromatherapy emerged and was embraced as an alternative medicine for many medical

[a] Mayo Clinic Hospital, Apheresis Department, 5777E Mayo Boulevard, Phoenix, AZ 85054, USA; [b] Austin Peay State University, School of Nursing, McCord Building, Clarksville, TN 37043, USA
* Corresponding author.
E-mail address: farrarf@apsu.edu

Nurs Clin N Am 55 (2020) 489–504
https://doi.org/10.1016/j.cnur.2020.06.015
0029-6465/20/Published by Elsevier Inc.

conditions. This article investigates the use of clinical aromatherapy. Credibility is seen in the historical evolution and nursing theorist support. Aromatherapy regulation of guidelines, plant sources for aromatic oils, and safe use of essential oils in symptom management in clinical aromatherapy is reviewed. Suggestions are recommended for a best practice model for clinical aromatherapy.

CLINICAL AROMATHERAPY

Aromatherapy is a fast-growing complementary therapy worldwide. According to the National Institutes of Health National Center for Complementary and Integrative Health, Americans spend more than $30.2 billion annually on this therapy.[1] It is predicted the global market will grow in spending to $5 trillion by 2050.[2] Aromatherapy also is called integrative medicine.[3] It is especially important for frontline nurses to understand the difference between alternative therapy and integrative therapy. In alternative medicine, the therapy works as an addition to conventional medical treatment, whereas integrative therapy is solo and replaces any conventional medical care. The National Institutes of Health National Center for Complementary and Integrative Health developed categories for these therapies—mind-body therapy, biologically based practices, manipulative and body-based practices, energy medicine, and whole medical systems, such as Ayurvedic medicine and traditional Chinese medicine.[3,4] Nursing health care aromatherapy falls into the category of mind-body therapy. Nursing health care uses essential oils to complement therapeutic interventions, decrease anxiety. It is expected that the plant-based essential oil applications can be measured, such as a preanxiety symptoms, interventions with essential oil, and postanxiety symptoms. The outcome from the administration of essential oil can be measured with a pre anxiety level and post level of anxiety to determine if the essential oil is effective.[4,5]

WORLDWIDE HISTORICAL EVOLUTION OF AROMATHERAPY

Aromatherapy has been used for thousands of years. Hippocrates, father of modern medicine, advocated the use of aromatherapy due to his belief that aromatic baths and scented massage were key to good health. Essential oils leaders emerged, supporting aromatherapy as a credible therapy for mind, body, and spirit. **Table 1** summarizes major historical timelines of countries and cultural influences, validating aromatherapy as medical, clinical, and holistic.

NURSING THEORISTS SUPPORT FOR HEALTH CARE AROMATHERAPY

Historical evolution of medical, clinical, and holistic uses of essential oils is embraced by 8 major nursing theorists. Their theoretic frameworks and concepts reflect the use of clinical aromatherapy as a patient-centered and holistic approach for balancing physical health, spiritual needs and well-being. The 8 theorists' embracement confirms health care aromatherapy is a credible alternative method (**Table 2**).

REGULATION GUIDELINES FOR ESSENTIAL OILS

The Food and Drug Administration (FDA) of the United States guidelines classify essential oils for aromatherapy as cosmetics, because they are not drugs for treating or prevention of a disease.[10] Therefore, aromatherapy essential oils are not regulated by the FDA. The US Consumer Product Safety Commission (CPSC) monitors unsafe products.[11] The CSPC enforces federal laws to protect consumers against unreasonable injury and death from products.[12] The following are examples of how these 2 federal organizations monitor essential oils.

Table 1
Historical evolution

Country	Cultural Therapy
Egyptian culture	Resins, balms, and fragrant oils Papyrus Ebers wrote a famous manuscript about aromatic medicine. This is believed to be around 2800 BC.
Iraq	A skeleton was found 30,000 years ago with concentration of extracted plant essential oils.
India	The Ayurveda natural system of medicine was based on disease due to an imbalance of stress in a person's consciousness. Need to regain balance by internal purifications followed by special diet, herbal remedies, massage therapy, yoga, and meditation
China	Shen Nung's manuscript listed 350 plants in 2800 BC. Ayurvedic physicians are called holy men. Indian shamans are known as perfumeros, from scents of plants. Chinese culture still embraces herbal medicine. Traditional Chinese medicine Based on harmony energy of yin-yang Opposites balance is key to health. Imbalance have illness Acupuncture, cupping, herbal teas, powders from plants, meditation, and herbal burning near skin
Greece	Theophrastus inherited the botanic garden from Aristotle. He wrote a book about specific uses and formulas for aromatics. Kyphi formula contained 16 plants and was used for sleep and anxiety, to soothe skin, and as an antidote for snake bite. He became the father of botany. Hippocrates wrote about aromatic baths and antibacterial properties and urged people to carry aromatic plants for protection. Pedanius Dioscorides wrote *De Materia Medica* covering 700 plants, including aromatics. Pre-Christian era emerged with the belief that essential oils were pagan. In response, Pope Gregory the Great passed a law banning all aromatics. Works of Galen and Hippocrates were smuggled to Syria for safekeeping.
Arabia	Ibn Sina, an Arabic physician, used aromatics, such as senna, camphor, and cloves, for medical treatment. Inhaled henbane was used as anesthetic. Topical sugar was used to stop bleeding. Rose or orange blossom was used as flavor to medicine. This led to the manufacturing of medicine. Medical aromatherapy emerged in the third century. The first private apothecary shop opened in Baghdad. with dispensing medicines. such as tinctures, suppositories, inhalants, and pills.
German	Hieronymus Braunschweig a surgeon and botanist, wrote a book on distillation of oils from plants that included 25 oils
France	In 1919, Gattefossé, a famous chemist, was burned in an explosion in his laboratory. The wounds became infected. Wound rinsing with essential oils eradicated the infection. He coined the term, aromatherapy, and was known for the medical use of essential oils with their antibacterial and healing properties of essential oils. Jean Valnet, an army physician, wrote the first aromatherapy book by a doctor. Shirley Price authored *Aromatherapy for Healthcare Professionals*. She is known for clinical use of essential oils. In 1961, Marguerite Maury, a nurse, published *Le Capital "Jeunesse"*. This book classified clinical departments' use of essential oils, such as surgery and spa treatment. Maury won 2 international awards for her research.

Table from Refs.[4–9]

Table 2 Nursing theoretic frameworks for health care aromatherapy	
Theorist Name	**Application to Clinical Practice**
Florence Nightingale Environmental	Cleanliness, rest, and relaxation properties
Myra Estrin Levine Holistic	Transformation process preventing stress
Hildegard Peplau Interpersonal relations	Supports interpersonal relations; promotes personal growth
Martha Rogers Unitary human beings and their environment are one	Interrelationship between people and plants
Sister Callista Roy Adaptation	Assist coping and adaptation
Wanda de Aguilar Horta Basic human needs	Restore balance, thereby decreasing depression and stress
	Promote holistic patient comfort
Jean Watson Transpersonal care	Holistic harmony caring interactive healing relationship such as massage and talk

Table from Ref.[4]

1. Aromatherapy waterless vaporizers and diffusers were recalled due to a defective heater causing a fire multiple times with consumers. The CPSC had the authority to cease the sale of the products and refund consumers.[11]
2. The FDA protects consumers from false claims and mislabeled products that mislead the public. Surveillance found Quinessence Aromatherapy Ltd posted on their website advertisement that essential oils protect against and cure coronavirus disease-2019. (COVID-19). This false statement triggered a FDA letter warning to the owner to take the information off their website within 48 hours and cease the sale of essential oil for prevention and cure of COVID-19. These 48 hours included developing a plan to be approved by the COVID-19 Task Force. The company was located in Europe with essential oils sold in the United States. The owner ignored the warning. Due to the fraudulent statement describing essential oils as a curing drug for COVID -19, a second joint letter was sent to the owner by the FDA, CPSC, the secretary of Health and Human Services, and the U.S. Public Health Services ordered the owner of the company to immediately take down the website and cease the sell of essential oils as a curing drug. The company's website was also put on the federal surveillance website list.

Administrators were ordered to cease sale and remove from the Web site immediately. This incidence of a false claim has brought awareness that currently essential oils are complementary therapy and do not treat and/or prevent a disease. Sellers need to be aware of descriptions of aromatherapy and consumers need to know that aromatherapy is complementary.[12]

NURSE AWARENESS OF ESSENTIAL OILS PLANT SOURCES AND USES

Essential oils are used every day for their aromatic scents—for example, perfumes, candles, essential oil plug-ins, scented aerosol sprays for the home, fabric softeners for clothes, hair shampoos, and spices to add flavor to food. Essential oils also are used in over-the-counter herbs and added to medications to add a pleasant flavor to bitter medications. These aromatic essential oils are growing in popularity, with nurses needing to learn about essential oils, their benefits, and safety measures. Essential oils come from seeds, stems, leaves, needles, petals, flowers, rinds and fruits, woods and resins, roots and rhizomes, and grasses. Oil is extracted from the plant by distillation by steam or mechanical cold press. Cher Kaufman, a certified aromatherapist, wrote a book with a series of chapters on plant sources for aromatic essential oils — seeds, petals and flowers, rinds and fruits, woods and resins, roots and rhizomes, and grass. The following is a summary of the plant sources of each category, with examples that could be significant to health care nurses.

Seeds

Three common examples of essential oils that come from seeds from plants are

1. Cardamom (*Ellettaria cardamomum*)—the essential oil is from the plant family Zingiberaceae. Uses for this seed oil include an antibacterial, antifungal, antispasmodic, aphrodisiac, digestive stimulant, expectorant, parasympathetic nervous system stimulant, and stimulant, tonic.
2. Black pepper *(Piper nigrum)* is from the plant family Piperaceae. Uses for this oil include an analgesic, antiseptic, antispasmodic, antitoxic, aphrodisiac, digestive, and circulatory tonic; reducing fever reducing pain; as a rubefacient; and for stimulating.
3. Sweet fennel (*Foeniculum vulgare* var. *dulce*) is from the plant family Apiaceae. Uses for this oil include an anti-inflammatory, antibacterial, antifungal, antispasmodic, detoxifier, and digestive and for relieving gas.[13]

Stems, Leaves, and Needles

There are 7 common examples of essential oils derived from stems, leaves, and needles.

1. Cistus (*Cistus ladanifer*) is from the plant family Cistaceae. This essential oil comes from stems, twigs, dried leaves, and dried flowers. Uses for this oil include as a cictrisant or for cell regeneration; as an antibacterial, anti-infectious, antimicrobial, astringent, and antiviral agent; as an immunity booster and regulator; as a tonic and support for parasympathetic and central nervous systems; and for wound healing.
2. Eucalyptus is a tree from the plant family Myrtaceae. It also is referred to by many names, such eucalyptus oil, blue gum oil, blue mallee oil, and gully gum oil. The leaves and twigs are used for burns, wounds, nasal congestion, lowering blood glucose, nasal congestion, and asthma and as a tick repellent. It also is used in medications and supplements.
3. Laurel (*Laurus nobilis*) is from the plant family Lauraceae. This aromatic evergreen scrub is known for its aromatic dark green, glossy leaves. Dried and fresh leaves oil is used as an analgesic, antibacterial, antimicrobial, antiseptic, antispasmodic, and antiviral; for boosting the immune system and calming the nervous system; and as an expectorant and fungicide.
4. Patchouli (*Pogostemon cablin*) comes from the plant family Lamiaceae that is commonly called the mint or dead needle busy herb. Oil from leaves are used as an antidepressant, anti-inflammatory, antimicrobial, antiviral, aphrodisiac, astringent, deodorant, and digestive; for relieving gas soothing the nervous system; and as a stimulant and tonic.

5. Peppermint (*Mentha x piperita* L) comes from the plant family Lamiacae in the mint family. Peppermint essential oil is a common flavoring agent in pharmaceuticals, soaps, cosmetics, food, and beverages. This essential is used as an analgesic, antibacterial, anti-inflammatory, antispasmodic, antimicrobial, decongestive, digestive, and expectorant and relieves coughs.
6. Pine (*Pinus sylvestris*)—pinus edulis is from the plant family Lamiaceae and from the mint family. Pine essential oil is derived from the needles on the pine tree. The scent is known for the uplifting and positive impact on the mood. It is known for treatment of postsurgery nausea and vomiting. Essential pine oil is used as an analgesic, anti-bacterial, antibiotic, anti-infectious, anti-inflammatory, antifungal, and antimicrobial agent; assisting in opening lungs and air pathways; as an expectorant; and for soothing nerves.
7. Rosemary (*Rosmarinus officinalis*) is from the plant family Lamiaceae. This aromatic evergreen shrub's essential oil is derived from leaves, flowers, and stems. This essential oil is known for folk medicine, flavoring food, and herbal tea. Rosemary has been known as a sacred oil. Uses for this essential oil are as an analgesic, anti-inflammatory, anti-infectious, antiseptic, and antispasmodic agent; for breaking up mucus; as a cognitive stimulant, decongestant, expectorant, muscle relaxant (cineole), stimulant, and tonic; and for wound healing (verbenone).[14]

Petal and Flowers

There are 8 common essential oils derived from petal and flowers.

1. Clary sage (*Salivia sclarea*) is an herbaceous perennial in the plant family Lamia-ceae with a history of petal and flowers used as an herb. The essential oil of clary sage is used in perfumes and muscatel flavoring in wines and liqueur. This essential oil is used as an antidepressant, antifungal, anti-inflammatory, antispasmodic, and aphrodisiac and for calming the nervous system, relaxing the uterus, and stimulating the blood flow.
2. Chamomile *(Matricaria chamomilla [Anthemis nobilis])* is in the plant family Astera-ceae and is a common name for several daisy-like flowers. Chamomile essential oil from flowers is used in herbal tea and is a popular night herbal tea due to the sedative affect. This essential oil is used for support for the nervous system, inflammation, insomnia, menstrual issues, headaches, and skin concerns.
3. Geranium (*Pelargonium x asperum*) and rose (*Pelargonium graveolent*)—this essential oil comes from the plant family Geraniaceae. This perennial plant has a sweet floral scent with uses in high-end perfumes and skin products with essentials oils resulting in young radiant skin. Essential oil from the flowers are used for reducing anxiety, as a sedative, for stimulating relaxation, as aids in symptoms from menstruation, as an anti-inflammatory, and for supporting healthy lymph drainage.
4. Jasmine (*Jasminum sambac*; *Jasminum grandiflorum*)—this essential oil is from the plant family Oleaceae. Jasmine is a genus of shrubs and vines in the olive family. Flowers of this bushy strong-scented perennial plant are used for scent and in tea as a base for green and white teas. As an essential oil, jasmine is used as an antidepressant and aphrodisiac, for calming the nervous system, and as a sexual tonic and stimulant.
5. Lavender (*Lavandula angustifolia*) —this essential oil is in the plant family of Lamia-ceae and is a bushy strong-scented perennial plant. Lavender is a popular house décor and frequently used with dried flowers as a complement in weddings. The popular scent is used in balms, salves, and cosmetics. As an essential oil, lavender is used as analgesic, anti-inflammatory, antifungal, and antispasmodic; for calming

the nervous system, lowering blood pressure, and reducing anxiety and sensations of pain; as a sedative; and for wound healing.

6. Neroli (*Citrus aurantium* var. *amara*)—this essential oil is in the plant family Rutaceae and is from the bitter orange tree. This essential oil from flowers has a rich floral scent and is known as orange blossom oil. Neroli is used in scented products, such as perfumes and lotions. This essential oil is used as an antidepressant, antifungal, anti-inflammatory, antimicrobial, antioxidant, antiparasitic, antiseptic, and aphrodisiac; for calming; and as a digestive, nervous system stimulant, sedative, and tonic.

7. Rose (*Rosa damascena; R damascena* var. *alba*)—this essential is from the plant family Lamiaceae and is a flowering shrub known as a rosebush. Rose oil is a powerful rich sweet smell. It is used commonly in perfumery. This essential oil is used as an antibacterial, antidepressant, anti-infectious, anti-inflammatory, antiseptic, antiviral, aphrodisiac, and astringent agent; for calming the nervous system and reducing anxiety; as a sedative; as a sexual, general, and uterine tonic; and for wound healing.

8. Ylang-ylang *(Cananga odorata)*—this essential oil is from the plant family Annonaceae, or custard apple family. This tropical flower is a yellow-shaped flower that grows on the cananga tree. Oil from ylang-ylang is used in cologne, lotion, food flavoring, and soap. This essential oil elevates the mood. Ylang-ylang essential oil is used as an antidepressant, anti-inflammatory, antiparasitic, antispasmodic, and aphrodisiac; for calming the nervous system and lowering blood pressure; and as a sexual tonic.[15]

Rinds and Fruits

1. Bergamot (*Citrus bergamia*) is from the plant family Rutaceae. This yellow or green fruit is a hybrid of lemon and bitter orange and has a bitter taste that is more than grapefruit but less than a lemon. The essential oil from the peel or zest of the fruit can cause photosensitivity, with sun exposure causing damage to sun-exposed skin. The essential oil has a citrus fruit smell, with uses in oil perfumes, cosmetics, and scenting food. This essential oil is used as an air purifier, antibacterial, antidepressant, antifungal, anti-inflammatory, and antiviral; for calming; as a deodorant; for digestive regulating (undereating or overeating); for reducing anxiety; as a sedative and tonic; and for wound healing.   .

2. Lemon (*citrus limonum*)—this essential oil is fruit from a small evergreen tree. This oil is from the Rutaceae plant family, with the peel of the fruit and pulp used in culinary and noncultural from lemon essential oil, lemon pie for culinary to cleaning products. The distinct sour taste of lemon is a popular essential oil. The essential oil from lemon is used as an antibacterial, anticoagulant, antidepressant, anti-infectious, anti-inflammatory, antiseptic, antiviral, astringent, antioxidant, and antimicrobial agent; as a digestive stimulant, immunity booster, and lymphatic; and for reducing anxiety.

3. Mandarin (*Citrus reticulata*) —this essential oil is from the Rutaceae plant family. This small citrus tree grows mandarin oranges that are smaller than oranges. A hybrid of the mandarin orange is the tangerine. The mandarin essential oil from peel and rind is sweeter and can be dried for seasoning and used in various food. This essential oil is used as an analgesic, antidepressant, antiseptic, central nervous system tonic, deodorant, digestive tonic, and immunity booster; for reducing reduces anxiety and fevers; and as a sedative.

4. Sweet orange *(citrus sinensis)*—this essential oil is from the plant family Rutaceae. This sweet citrusy greenish orange fruit oil is from the peel and zest. This oil is used

in top perfumes. The leaves are photosensitive but not the fruit. The sweet orange essential oil is used as an analgesic, antidepressant, antibacterial antifungal, antiseptic, antiviral, deodorant, and digestive tonic; for reducing anxiety; as a sedative; for soothing the nervous system; and as a stimulant.

5. Juniper berry (*Juniperus communis*)—this purple-black berry is a female evergreen cone. This essential oil is from the plant family Cupressaceae, derived from conifers, and often is used as a spice. The essential oil is used as an analgesic, antiseptic, antiseborrheic, anti-inflammatory, antifungal, antiviral, decongestant, and detoxifier and for increasing circulation and reducing fever.[16]

Woods and Resins

1. Cedarwood (*Cedrus atlantica*)—cedarwood is from the plant family Pinaceae and the needles, leaves, bark, and wood are for extracting the essential oil. The evergreen conifers have a soothing woodsy scent. The essential oil is used as an antifungal, antiseptic, and astringent; for breaking up mucus; and as a calmative, insect repellent, lymphatic decongestant, and general tonic.
2. Frankincense (*Boswellia carteri*)—this essential oil is in the plant family of Burseraceae and is from a Boswellia tree. Resin that is a hardened gumlike material is used in aromatic incense and perfumes. The essential oil is used as an analgesic, antibacterial, antidepressant, anti-infectious, antimicrobial, and astringent agent; for immunity tonic; for reducing anxiety; as a sedative; and for soothing the nervous system and wound healing.
3. Sandalwood (*Santalum album*)—this essential oil is from the plant family Santalaceae. The oil is extracted from wood, heartwood of the trunk, and sawdust. The essential oil from sandalwood is used in medications, skin beauty treatment, incense sticks, perfumes, mouthwashes, deodorants, and antiseptics. As an essential oil, it is used as an antibacterial, antidepressant, anti-inflammatory, antimicrobial, antiviral, aphrodisiac, and sedative; for soothing the soothes nervous system; and as a general tonic.[17]

Roots and Rhizomes

1. Ginger (*Zingiber officinale*) is distilled from the rhizome or underground stem of a root of the herb zingiber. Ginger also is known as the oil of empowerment for the feeling of confidence. Ginger root oil is a frequently used spice. In addition, this dried and ugly root is used as an analgesic, antibacterial, antispasmodic, digestive support, immunity harmonizer, and rubefacient.
2. Vetiver (*Vetiveria zizanoides*) is derived from the aromatic roots and also called khus oil. It is derived from the vetiver plant that is a clumpy, green grass that can grow 5 feet or more. This essential oil is used as an antiseptic, antispasmodic, anti-inflammatory, digestive stimulant, immunity booster, and sedative, and for skin support and soothing the nervous system.[18]

Grass

1. Lemongrass (*Cymbopogon citratus*) is an essential oil that comes from the leaves and stalk of the lemongrass plant. This grassy plant is used in cooking and herbal tea. The oil from the grass has a lemony powerful scent and is bright or pale yellow. This essential oil is used as an analgesic, antidepressant, antiviral, immunity booster, and general tonic.
2. Palmarosa (*Cymbopogon martinii* var. *motia*) is an essential oil that comes from a tall herbaceous grass and can be called Indian geranium or rose oil. The oil has a sweet citrus lemony scent that has a yellow color.[19]

ADMINISTRATION OF ESSENTIAL OILS

There are 4 basic methods for administration of essential oils. Nursing commonly uses topical skin application of essential oil for administration. If a facility has an integrative medicine department, massage therapy usually includes an essential oil. The following is an overview of the 4 methods by which essential oils are absorbed.

1. Topical application with skin absorption of the essential oil. Examples include massage, scented bath, cosmetics, and perfumes.
2. Absorption of the essential oil by inhaling in nostrils. Examples include direct inhalation via diffuser with steam, aroma stones, and oil-scented strip of cloth. Indirect absorption examples include scented room spray and heated candle wax, detergent, and bathroom and floor cleaners.
3. Oral absorption of the essential oil. Examples include gelatin capsules and safe dose of essential oil diluted.
4. Internal absorption of essential oil. Examples include scented mouthwash and scented suppository or vagina douche. Essential oil used for flavor in prescription medications and herbal medicines.[20–22]

PATHOPHYSIOLOGIC RESPONSE TO HEALTH CARE AROMATHERAPY

When essential oil in aromatherapy is inhaled, molecules activate the olfactory, respiratory, gastrointestinal, and/or integumentary systems based on the pathway of activation. These molecules are capable of releasing neurotransmitters, such as endorphins, to trigger a sense of well-being and an analgesic effect.[20,21] There are 2 common pathways triggering a pathophysiologic response to aromatherapy molecules. The most common pathway is inhalation, such as by a diffuser. Activation of olfactory stimulation produces immediate change in parameters for blood pressure, pulse rate, muscle tension, pupil dilation, body temperature, and blood flow.[20,21] The following summarizes this pathway:

- The olfactory stimulation by aromatherapy travels via nostrils to the olfactory bulb.
- The stimulus then travels to the brain for processing, where the amygdala triggers an emotional response and the hippocampus retrieves and/or forms memories.
- The limbic system interacts with the cerebral cortex, activating thoughts and feelings.
- The inhaled aromatherapy molecules travel to the upper respiratory tract and then to the lower respiratory tract.
- Molecules than travel to the pulmonary blood vessels to the blood stream then to organs and tissues.[20,21]
- In summary, the inhaled aromatherapy molecules affect mind, body, and spirit.

The second common pathway is through the skin, such as by a massage, in which molecules are absorbed through the skin. The pathway is summarized:

- The molecules travel to the upper respiratory track and then the lower respiratory tract.
- Molecules then travel to the pulmonary blood vessels, to the blood stream, and then to organs and tissues.[20,21]
- The skin pathway can activate olfactory stimulation and also activates application of scented oil to the skin pathway triggering a mental and physiological response.

- The skin pathway absorption of essential oils can reduce a patient's perceived stress, enhance healing, and increase communication.[20]

SAFE USE OF ESSENTIAL OILS

Coming home from a long challenging day of work to the aromatic smell of a favorite essential oil can immediately decrease the stress from a busy and challenging day. Relaxing in a scented uplifting bubble bath can make someone feel like a new person. On the flip side, aromatic essential oils can be toxic, causing chemical burns and even death. Aromatherapy is growing in usage and can be extremely dangerous if not used safely because of a knowledge deficit. Two ethical principles apply to nurses when administering essential oils. The first is beneficence, in which the nurse takes positive steps to prevent harm. The second ethical principle is nonmaleficence, which means having an obligation to do no harm to a patient. Legal consequences could result if harm to a patient occurs due to negligence from administering of aromatherapy. Therefore, the bottom line is the need for nurses to learn about aromatherapy essential oils and their potential harms, such as poison and lethal complication. The following case reports portray safety considerations, complications, and interventions.

Combustion Reaction Safety

TF is a 54-year-old man who lives in Phoenix, Arizona; he is an advocate of essential oils and frequently uses them for anxiety and to promote sleep. On his day off, TF has several errands, including his monthly supply of essential oils. His first errand was to purchase essential oils. During his last errand, TF heard his name being called by an old friend. TF sat down to visit with his friend for a few minutes; the visit lasted 45 minutes. When TF returned to his car, he found black smoke in the car and a large burnt hole in his backseat where his purchased essential oils were placed. TF called the police to file a report.

Critical analysis revealed the large supply of essential oils were stored in the back seat. TF left the oils in the car for 45 minutes with the outside temperature of 112°F, with the potential increase in the temperature in the car increasing to 160°F. The essential oils caught on fire, resulting in the smoke and burnt hole in the backseat of the car.

Intervention for this unsafe use of essential oil is education that these oils are flammable and need to be stored in a cool dark place in the original bottle, which is colored to prevent direct sunlight penetrating to the essential oil. Unsafe storage by leaving essential oils in a hot car can cause a combustion reaction, triggering flames and a fire.

Elder and Child Safety

CF, a 66-year-old woman, was admitted for inpatient treatment of sepsis from an acute urinary infection. At night she can become agitated and screamed that snakes were crawling up her wall. The provider ordered aromatherapy and increased lighting in the room. Turning on a bed alarm and increased rounding also were ordered. The nurse brought the aromatherapy essential oil to the room and left to get a steam diffuser. When the nurse returned, CF appeared drunk. The nurse found the bottle open on the bedside table. The nurse called for assistance.

Critical analysis revealed the nurse left the bottle of essential oil on the nightstand unattended when she left the room. The patient was able to open the bottle and drink a small amount of the essential oil, causing the drunken behavior.

Intervention for essential oil left attended with a confused elderly patient was administration of milk to dilute the essential oil. The provider was called for further orders and an incident report was completed. The elderly and children are vulnerable to adverse effects from inappropriate use of essential oils. Early recognition is appearing drunk. Essential oils should be locked in a container in a hospital and kept away from elders and children. An essential oil bottle should not be left unattended, especially with this confused patient with delusions. The diffuser with the essential oil needs to be prepared outside of the patient's room.[11]

Allergic Contact Dermatitis and Primary Contact Dermatitis

TA, a 30-year-old woman, works at a massage therapist and is extremely popular. Bookings must be in advance because her schedule stays full. Each day she works 8 hours to 9 hours, with mostly 1.5-hour massages. She uses a lotion with an aromatic essential oil. After 3 months, she developed a bright bred rash on her hands and lower arms. She used a steroid cream on the rash without resolving the rash. Over the next month, the rash got worse. TA scheduled an appointment with a dermatologist.

Critical analysis evaluated allergic contact dermatitis versus primary contact dermatitis. In allergic contact dermatitis, the allergy occurs over a period whereas primary contact dermatitis occurs the first time the essential oil is used. In allergic contact dermatitis, the symptoms are a bright red rash that worsens with time whereas the primary contact dermatitis a presents as a red wheal or burn.[20,23]

Intervention was based on treating allergic contact dermatitis based on symptomatology and length of time. Patch testing revealed the specific essential oil to stop using, allowing her to continue as a massage therapist. If TA had primary contact dermatitis, the red wheal or burn area from the toxic oil would be diluted with vegetable oil or milk then washed with unscented soap.[23]

Essential Oil Phototoxicity

AJ is a 34-year-old woman who loves the sun. She lives in an apartment with a swimming pool. The average summer temperature is 102°F. On weekends she can be found at the swimming pool for 4 hours per weekend day. AJ's pool relaxing is 4 hours to 5 hours per day. She sets an alarm hourly to turn from back to stomach. AJ says the sunrays lift her up and gives her a beautiful brown tan with sunscreen oil. Due to the shutdown of her state due to COVID-19 and stores closed, AJ decided to shop online for home delivery of essential oils. AJ found a Web site with a sale on essential oils that had a pop-up advertisement declaring breaking news that essential oils prevent and cure the COVID-19 virus. AJ purchased several citrus fruit essential oils. AJ applied a mandarin essential oil to her neck and chest to ward off the COVID-19 virus. AJ left the pool early because of a burning sensation on her neck and chest. She took a shower and noticed several burned areas. The next day, the red burned areas turned to a brown skin damage appearance unlike any sunburn she ever experienced. AJ scheduled a dermatologist appointment due to the discoloration and discomfort not resolving.[16,20,23]

Critical analysis revealed that AJ was scammed by a fraudulent online statement to sell essential oils in a pandemic COVID-19 fearful time. The mandarin essential oil was not diluted when applied to the skin, increasing the risk for dermal toxicity. The pure mandarin essential oil was phototoxic and inflected damage to the skin, resulting in dark pigmented skin that could be permanent.[16,23] Dermal toxicity also occurred with the essential oil not being diluted. The regular sunburn resulted in redness and blisters on her skin. AJ scheduled an urgent dermatology appointment. She used an over-the-counter steroid cream for pain relief.

The intervention to stop using the phototoxic essential oil and seek a specialist, which AJ did, with scheduling the dermatology appointment. The essential oil label always should be read for safety instructions. If a photosensitivity essential oil is used, wait a minimum of 12 hours before exposure to sun ultraviolet radiation. AJ should consult a qualified aromatherapist who has training for aromatherapy, not a seller of essential oils, to prevent harm from essential oils. A registry database for trained aromatherapists who have passed the core level of aromatherapy examination can be found at thttps://www.aromatherapycouncil.org.uk/about_us [10] Essential oils always should be diluted in a carrier oil. A carrier oil prevents irritation to the skin and side effects of the essential oil. Examples of carrier oils include coconut oil, coconut oil, aloe vera gel, unscented lotion, vegetable oil, and avocado oil. Because oil and water do not mix, milk is used to remove the oil and calm the skin followed by washing of the skin by unscented soap.[23]

Phototoxic essential oil contains constituents that triggers a chemical process that changes the skin DNA, making the skin susceptible to sun ultraviolet radiation. This chemical change in the skin is called photosensitivity and the primary constituent is confurocoumarins that causes phototoxic reaction. Exposure of the applied photosensitivity essential oil to ultraviolet radiation from the sun inflicts skin damage with darkly pigmented skin that can be permanent due to the long period of exposure to sun ultraviolet radiation.[23] It is extremely important to determine if an essential oil is phototoxic. AJ should find this warning on the label of the essential oil. Essential oils are not regulated by the FDA but the FDA monitors Web sites for fraudulent postings. AJ should report the online site and harm to her skin to the FDA for investigation.[11]

Oral Toxicity

LM, a 110-pounds 20-year-old woman who lived with her mother, was told by an essential oil seller that she heard essential oils could prevent and cure COVID-19. LM was terrified that she could contract the virus with a resurgence of COVID-19 later in the year. LM was extremely excited about this information and asked which essential oil she should use orally to protect herself from this deadly pandemic COVID-19 virus. The seller recommended a safe dose for eucalyptus essential oil twice weekly orally. After a week LM decided to increase the oral dose to ward off the COVID-19 virus. She decided to drink half of an 8 oz glass of eucalyptus essential oil. Within 10 minutes she experienced burning in her throat, mouth, and stomach.[23] LM yelled for her mother to come quickly. The mother found the daughter vomiting, staggering, and with slurred speech. The mother found the eucalyptus essential oil bottle and a glass indicating she had drunk eucalyptus essential oil. The mother called 911 with the dispatcher sending an ambulance and notifying the Poison Control Center for eucalyptus poisoning.

Critical analysis of oral toxicity of eucalyptus revealed LM had drunk an unsafe dose causing poisoning with central nervous system depression and a chemical burn in her mouth, throat, and stomach. LM was admitted to the intensive care unit.

Intervention was police investigation of the fraudulent information that eucalyptus could prevent and cure COVID-19 information by the seller of the essential oil with unintentional poisoning LM. A qualified aromatherapist that is certified or completed aromatherapy curriculum. Don't take advise from a seller of essential oils without expertise. Seek consultation for safe use of essential oils.[11] Even with a safe oral dose of eucalyptus can cause harm. Safe use of essential oils is to not take essential oils internally. It is extremely important that induced vomiting is not done for this toxicity.

Oral toxicity symptoms are rapid decline with complaint of burning in the mouth and throat and abdominal pain. Central nervous symptoms are ataxia and respiratory depression, and, with a higher dose, possible nasal intubation is needed for mechanical ventilation and deep coma. Death can occur with a toxic dose.[20,23]

Eye Safety

MF accidently splashed essential oil in an eye when she was preparing essential oil for a diffuser. Her eye was burning and painful and her vision blurred in the eye.

Critical analysis reveals essential oils are toxic to eyes and can result in a chemical burn. The eye should be rapidly irrigated with milk or a vegetable oil carrier. A washcloth or cotton ball can help with the irrigation. After treatment flush the eye with water. Do not flush the eye with water initially due to oil and water not mixing.

AROMATHERAPY CLINICAL MANAGEMENT

Clinical nursing aromatherapy is patient symptom management with measuring the outcome in a clinical setting. When aromatherapy is ordered by a provider for symptom management, a nurse needs to perform a history assessment, obtain vital signs, identify the symptom, educate the patient, measure symptom management, evaluate the effectiveness, and document the plan of care.[1,6,7,24] The following is an overview of clinical management of the essential oil:

- Allergy—inhalant, skin, food, and medication allergy or sensitivity. Consider the need for a patch test.
- Chronic conditions—assess condition that could be impacted by aromatherapy, such as plant source triggering asthma attack or cancer that is fed by estrogen, with a few essential oils having estrogenic activity.
- Obtain vital signs—assess if there is a problem proceeding with essential oil administration.
- Symptoms needing to be managed—such as anxiety, depression, insomnia, nausea, and pain
- Educate the patient about the essential oil, procedure, safety, symptom management, patient-centered selection of the essential oil, and consent for implementation.
- Outcome measurement of symptom relief—select a tool for measuring the symptom, such as pain. The pain tool could be measurement of pain from 1 to 10 or visual picture rating of pain; or, a nonverbal patient's pain could be measured with a visual picture range, and pain in a patient unable to communicate could be measured with physiologic changes, such as vital signs, guarding of the area, and facial grimaces from discomfort. After selection of the pain measurement tool, rate the presymptom range, and post-implementation, measure at end of post symptom score for a change in outcome findings.
- Evaluate the effectiveness of the essential oil on the symptom. The outcome goals are decrease in the symptom and increased well-being and quality of life. Patient-centered symptom management and presence of a nurse could increase patient satisfaction.
- Document the procedure and incorporate into the plan of care.
- Examples of clinical conditions and settings that can benefit in the management of symptoms in the inpatient and outpatient settings are pain, nausea and vomiting, preoperative anxiety, critical care, general well-being, anxiety, depression, stress, insomnia, respiratory, dementia, oncology, palliative care, hospice, and end of life.[1,6,7,24]

BEST PRACTICE MODEL FOR CLINICAL SYMPTOM MANAGEMENT

Aromatherapy is used as an alternative medicine and complement to traditional care. Aromatherapy is rising in popularity and is a cost-effective symptom manager. The following are suggested steps for guidance and triggers for brainstorming to develop a customized patient-centered symptom management program using essential oils in an inpatient or outpatient setting.

1. Buy-in from major stakeholders. Develop a committee that includes interprofessional members. Input from all stakeholders, including frontline nurses, needs to be embraced; and, commit, by a recorded vote, to proceeding with the aromatherapy program.
2. Develop a policy and procedure manual. Search the literature for best practice aromatherapy models. If possible, contact the facility for assistance with the startup of the program. For example, a best practice model is at the Mayo Clinic in Phoenix Arizona. This research and education facility uses aromatherapy for alternative medicine and has integrative medicine.
3. Upon approval, establish guidelines for safe and effective implementation, including infection control, safe storage, and disposal of the chemical oil.
4. Identify common symptoms that could occur in the facility, such as pain, anxiety, depression, nausea, and insomnia.
5. Identify nursing considerations, such as assessment, chronic illness, administration, and safety.
6. Identify preoutcome and postoutcome measurements and best tools for measurement. For example, anxiety is a symptom: identify a pretest and post-test to measure anxiety that is a short tool.
7. Identify and educate aromatherapy champions to lead the new program by supervising and mentoring nurses, for example, a classroom course for hospital nurses and a certified clinical aromatherapy practitioner course.
8. Evaluate the data from the pre-intervention and post-intervention of aromatherapy. Interpret the findings and refine if needed.
9. Data analysis to justify aromatherapy is an effective intervention for symptom management.
   10. Seek a provider standing order for aromatherapy for sustainability.[1,24]

SUMMARY

Aromatic scents and oils used in clinical aromatherapy can be beneficial for symptom management such as pain, nausea, vomiting, anxiety, depression, stress, insomnia, agitation with dementia, cancer pain, and end of life symptoms, Clinical aromatherapy has been found beneficial in the inpatient and outpatient settings especially critical care, oncology, palliative care, hospice, and surgical. On the flip side, aromatic essential oils can be dangerous and toxic due to certain oils being flammable, causing skin dermatitis, or being phototoxic, with risks of chemical burn, oral toxicity, and even death. Therefore, it is important that nurses learn about essential oils. If a facility has a clinical aromatherapy program, it is critical that frontline nurses be educated with a classroom course on essential oils. Champions need to be selected for a clinical aromatherapy practitioner course. These certified aromatherapists can lead the program, serve as consultants, and mentor nurses.

DISCLOSURE

A.J. Farrar and F.C. Farrar have no commercial or financial conflicts of interest or any funding sources.

REFERENCES

1. Pace S. Essential Oils in Hospitals: The Ethics, Safety, Cost and Application of Clinical Aromatherapy. Available at: https://www.tisserandinstitute.org/essential-oils-in-hospitals/. Accessed March 30, 2020.
2. Swamy MK, Akgtar MS, Sinniah UR. Antimicrobial properties of plant essential oils against human pathogens and their mode of action: an updated review. evidence based complementary and alternative medicine. 2016. Available at: https://www.ncbi.nlm.nih.gov/pmc/articles/PMC5206475/. Accessed July 30, 2019.
3. National Center for Complementary and Integrative Health. Complementary, Alternative, or Integrative Health: What's in a Name? NCCIH Pub NO.: D347. Available at: http://www.nccih.nih.gov. Accessed April 4, 2020.
4. Gnatta JR, Kurebayashi LFS, Turrini RNT, et al. Aromatherapy and nursing: historical and theoretical conception. Rev Esc Enferm USP 2016;50(1):127–33.
5. Alliance of International Aromatherapists. AIA Journal. Aromatherapy. Available at: https://www.alliance-aromatherapists.org/history-basics. Accessed March 30, 2020.
6. PDQ Integrative, Alternatives, and Complementary Therapies Editorial Board. Aromatherapy with Essential Oils (PDQ)-Health Professional Version. Beethesda,MD: National Cancer Institute. Available at: https://www.cancer.gov/about-cancer/treatment/cam/hp/aromatherapy-pdq. Accessed March 30, 2020.
7. Aromatherapy HL, Lindquest R, Tracy MR, et al, editors. Complementary and alternative therapies in nursing. 8th edition. New York: Springer Publishing Company; 2018. p. 319–38.
8. Libster MM. Evolution of aromatherapy. In: Buckle J, editor. Clinical aromatherapy essential oils in healthcare. 3rd edition. St Louis (MO): Elsevier; 2015. p. 2–14.
9. National Association of Holistic Aromatherapists. What is Aroma Therapy? Available at: https://www.aromaweb.com/articles/wharoma.asp. Accessed March 30, 2020.
10. U.S. Food & Drug Administration. Aromatherapy. Available at: https://www.fda.gov/cosmetics/cosmetic-products/aromatherapy#essentialoil. Accessed March 30, 2020.
11. Consumer Product Safety Commission. Regulations, Laws & Standards. Available at: https://www.cpsc.gov/Regulations-Laws–Standards. Accessed April 20,2020.
12. Federal Trade Commission. Quinessence Aromatherapy LTD. Available at: https://www.ftc.gov/warning-letters/quinessence-aromatherapy-ltd. Accessed March 30,2020.
13. Kaufmann C. Chapter 8. Seeds. In: Nature's essential oils: aromatic alchemy for well-being. New York: The Country Man Press; 2018. p. 119–28.
14. Kaufmann C. Chapter 9. Stems, leaves, & needles in nature's essential oils: aromatic alchemy for well-being. New York: The Country Man Press; 2018. p. 129–50.
15. Kaufmann C. Chapter 10. Petals & flowers. In: Nature's essential oils: aromatic alchemy for well-being. New York: The Country Man Press; 2018. p. 151–76.

16. Kaufmann C. Chapter 11. Rinds & fruits in nature's essential oils: aromatic alchemy for well-being. New York: The Country Man Press; 2018. p. 177–94.
17. Kaufmann C. Chapter 12. Woods & resins. In: Nature's essential oils: aromatic alchemy for well-being. New York: The Country Man Press; 2018. p. 195–206.
18. Kaufmann C. Chapter 13. Roots & rhizomes. In: Nature's essential oils: aromatic alchemy for well-being. New York: The Country Man Press; 2018. p. 207–12.
19. Kaufmann C. Chapter 14. Grass. In: Nature's essential oils: aromatic alchemy for well-being. New York: The Country Man Press; 2018. p. 213–8.
20. National Association Holistic Aromatherapy. Exploring Aromatherapy. Available at: https://naha.org/explore-aromatherapy/about-aromatherapy/what-is-aromatherapy/. Accessed March 30, 2020.
21. Libster MM. How essentials work. In: Buckle J, editor. Clinical aromatherapy essential oils in healthcare. 3rd edition. St Louis (MO): Elsevier; 2015. p. 15–36.
22. International Federation of Aromatherapists What is Aromatherapy. Available at: https://ifaroma.org/en_GB/home/explore_aromatherapy/about-aromatherapy. Accessed March 30, 2020.
23. Libster MM. Toxicity & contraindications. In: Buckle J, editor. Clinical aromatherapy essential oils in healthcare. 3rd edition. St Louis (MO): Elsevier; 2015. p. 73–94.
24. Libster MM. Aromatherapy in integrative healthcare. In: Buckle J, editor. Clinical aromatherapy essential oils in healthcare. 3rd edition. St Louis (MO): Elsevier; 2015. p. 95–116.

Reiki, Nursing, and Health Care

Kathie Lipinski, MSN, RN[a,*], Jane Van De Velde, DNP, RN[b,1]

KEYWORDS

- Reiki and nursing • Complementary or integrative therapy • Self-care
- Reiki in hospitals • Reiki research • Reiki for self-care • Reiki volunteer programs

KEY POINTS

- Consumer demand is driving the integration of complementary and integrative health services such as Reiki into health care environments.
- Nurses can take leadership roles within their administrative and clinical settings to introduce complementary modalities such as Reiki to colleagues, patients, and families.
- Nurses can use Reiki for a self-care practice to manage the pressures faced in their day-to-day work environments and to prevent burnout and unhealthy coping.
- Reiki is safe, gentle, and easy to use, making it clinically appropriate for many types of patient care situations.
- Systematic reviews of current research report that Reiki shows promise in helping to increase relaxation; reduce pain, anxiety, and depression; and improve general well-being.

INTRODUCTION

The use of complementary and integrative health (CIH) services is increasing with more Americans seeking and using these modalities as an adjunct to routine medical care. These modalities include Reiki, acupuncture, massage, yoga, naturopathy, and meditation.[1] These are health care approaches that have origins outside of customary Western practice and are not usually included in conventional medical care.[2]

However, it is possible for these nonmainstream practices to be integrated into standard health care regimens. When such practices are used together with conventional medicine, they are referred to as complementary health care.[2] When conventional and complementary practices are brought together in a coordinated way with a holistic, patient-focused approach to health care and wellness, it is classified as integrative health care.[2]

More than 800 hospitals (15%) in the United States currently offer Reiki services for patients.[3,4] A 2008 American Hospital Association (AHA) survey found that 84% of hospitals reported patient demand as the primary rationale in offering complementary

a Private Practice: Healing from the Heart NY; b Private Practice: The Reiki Share Project
1 Present address: P.O. Box 6983, Villa Park, IL 60181.
* Corresponding author. 224 Village Green Drive, Port Jefferson Station, NY 11776.
E-mail address: kathiekaruna95@aol.com

Nurs Clin N Am 55 (2020) 505–519
https://doi.org/10.1016/j.cnur.2020.06.018
0029-6465/20/© 2020 Elsevier Inc. All rights reserved.
nursing.theclinics.com

therapies, including Reiki.[5] A survey conducted in 2010 by Health Forum, a subsidiary of the AHA and Samueli Institute, reported similar results with the additional finding that 70% of the hospitals surveyed stated clinical effectiveness as their top reason for offering complementary therapies.[6] The survey results also reinforce the fact that patients want the best that both conventional medicine and complementary therapies can offer, and hospitals are responding.[6]

Why Nurses Are Important for Reiki

The World Health Organization (WHO) has designated 2020 as the Year of the Nurse and the Midwife in honor of the 200th anniversary of the birth of Florence Nightingale.[7] In an impressive 18-year running streak, Americans have rated nurses as the #1 most ethical and honest profession, according to the most recent annual Gallup poll.[8]

With this level of public trust, nurses are well positioned within their clinical settings to introduce complementary or integrative modalities such as Reiki to colleagues, patients, and families. Reiki is an excellent method of expressing compassionate concern for patients and clients through a caring presence, active listening, and gentle touch.[9] Nurses are witness to the pain, suffering, fear, and anxiety that their patients experience. Nurses who already know that Reiki can bring relaxation and healing to patients are in a prime position to weave Reiki into their routine care. Their daily work with patients gives them insight into additional areas of investigation for the use and effectiveness of Reiki.[10]

Reiki can maximize patient or client contact time because it makes the most of a few minutes of touch. It can help relieve stress, agitation, and acute or chronic pain. It can provide overall deep relaxation, helping patients to slip into sleep or, conversely, energize them when they are tired and depleted.[11]

It is important to understand that the use of Reiki is not simply an application of a treatment or intervention.[12] It is not one more thing that nurses have to do in their already hectic day. When someone offers Reiki, the receiver and the giver often feel as if they were entering a meditative, quiet, introspective state that allows both participants to become centered, relaxed, and fully present. It is a moment in time when nurses can refresh and clear the mind and reconnect with a quiet place within of peace and calmness.

When a nurse is fully present and available for a patient or a colleague in this quiet place, a Reiki treatment becomes a healing moment during which a deep connection with others honors the totality of who they are in body, mind, and spirit.

REIKI FOR SELF-CARE

With the many pressures and challenges that nurses currently face to provide quality nursing care in a complex and demanding health care environment, self-care is of utmost importance in managing stress and expanding coping skills. Many nurses struggle with balancing personal needs and the demands of the workplace and often find it challenging to set aside time for personally restorative practices.[13] "Reiki is unique among hands-on therapeutic modalities in its effectiveness in providing care to the caretaker."[13] It induces the calmness needed to stay focused and enhances inner resources.[14]

There are a variety of studies that have examined the effects of offering Reiki training to nurses for self-care purposes, in particular as a strategy to help them manage the pressures faced in their day-to-day work environments in order to prevent burnout and the creation of unhealthy coping mechanisms. In a study of nurses and Reiki practice, Cuneo and colleagues[15] found that the more nurses practiced self-Reiki, the more effective it was in supporting stress reduction. In addition, Deible and colleagues[16] found that nurses who practiced self-care techniques, including Reiki, were better able to cope with daily personal and work-related stressors in a healthy manner. Other findings revealed a significant increase in the presence of mindfulness as well as a lessening of job-related exhaustion for study participants.[16]

Diaz-Rodrigues and colleagues[17] found that a single 30-minute Reiki treatment could significantly relieve the negative effect of job stress in nurses diagnosed with burnout syndrome. They also suggested that Reiki treatments could be a cost-effective way to manage and prevent job stress for people at risk for burnout.[17]

The relationship between self-care and an improved ability to care for others was another important theme that emerged in several studies.[14,16,18] Taking the time for self-care with Reiki is an investment in nurses' overall well-being and may contribute to providing a higher quality of patient care.[4,15,16]

Caring for Self and Caring for Others

Connecting with Reiki for self-care is like being in a personal quiet space[14] not shared with anyone. Like meditation, self-Reiki can easily be woven into a nurse's daily life by spending 5 or 10 minutes doing Reiki throughout the day: in the morning on awakening or at bedtime, during a break at work, before or after working with a challenging patient, or in the office between clients. Focus and quiet are not always necessary because nurses can self-treat while sitting at a desk, during change of shift report, at a meeting, or when documenting.

The hectic pace of the health care profession is sometimes hard to avoid, and sharing Reiki in a health care setting is not limited to oneself or to patients. Nurses who practice Reiki can help to create a healing environment where they can support and nourish themselves and their colleagues wherever they work. Simply pausing and offering a few moments of Reiki can calm and relax staff, empowering them to better handle stressful situations and enhancing their ability to meet patient needs.

Code Lavender

Code Lavender is a rapid response tool used to support any person in a Cleveland Clinic hospital when patients, family members, or hospital staff are in crisis and in serious need of emotional support and care.[19] The concept was developed in 2008 as part of a holistic initiative[20] and is used "when challenging situations threaten unit stability, personal emotional equilibrium, or professional functioning."[19]

The Code Lavender team is an interdisciplinary team usually composed of holistically trained nurses and chaplains but can also include other hospital-based support services and volunteers. Once the code is called, members of the team respond within 30 minutes to offer support and holistic practices such as Reiki, meditation, and acupressure.[19] Johnson[20] reported in 2014 that 99.9% of all Code Lavenders are called to support hospital staff known as caregivers.

This holistic rapid response model weaves care for the caregivers into the workplace setting and sends the message that ongoing support is available.

REIKI IN HEALTH CARE ORGANIZATIONS

As complementary and integrative healing modalities are increasingly being introduced into health care organizations, in both inpatient and outpatient settings, patients and caregivers can receive the benefits of meditation, massage, yoga, acupuncture, biofeedback, and energy healing therapies.[1] Reiki, in particular, is gaining more acceptance as a healing practice. As noted earlier, 15% of the hospitals in the United States (>800 hospitals) offer Reiki services for patients.[3,4] Offering these additional healing modalities is an ideal way to emphasize the importance of patient-centered care[21,22] and an acknowledgment of the importance that institutions place on the patient experience.[23] These types of modalities can positively contribute to patients' and families' experiences across the spectrum of health care

Reiki Volunteer Programs

Reiki is often introduced into patient care areas through volunteer programs, with Reiki practitioners recruited from both in-house staff and the community. Hospitals have offered Reiki training programs to employees with the intent that they will integrate Reiki into their patient care activities. However, Hahn and colleagues[24] reported that in-house staff are often not available to offer Reiki sessions because of time constraints and multiple responsibilities in providing patient care. Volunteers can fill that gap for busy health care providers.

Nurses are often the ones who introduce energy-based modalities (EBMs)[12] into their workplaces. A few examples of nurses' involvement in establishing Reiki volunteer programs include the program at the Portsmouth Regional Hospital in New Hampshire,[25,26] founded in 1995 by Patricia Alandydy, RN; and the program at Hartford Hospital in Connecticut,[27] founded in 1998 with guidance from Alice Moore, RN.[28] Nurses were also key members of planning teams that founded Reiki volunteer programs at Brigham and Women's Hospital in Boston, Massachusetts,[24] and the Mayo Clinic in Minnesota.[29]

In these institutions, Reiki is being offered to patients throughout the system (eg, presurgical and postsurgical areas[25]; in intensive care units; medical, surgical, and obstetrics/gynecology floors; and outpatient cancer infusion centers). Staff also receive the benefits of Reiki sessions from volunteers. Hahn and colleagues[24] reported that emergency room staff at Brigham and Women's Hospital received Reiki sessions to help them cope with the stress of caring for victims of the 2013 Boston Marathon bombing.

Reiki in Hospitals Training Programs

Several comprehensive training programs have been developed to provide the knowledge and skills to prepare Reiki practitioners for working safely alongside health care professionals in hospitals and other medical settings. These programs are also dedicated to conducting research that examines the efficacy and impact of the use of Reiki in a medical setting. Practitioners are paid for their services once training is completed.

Medical Reiki™ (https://www.ravenkeyesmedicalreiki.com/), a program to train Reiki practitioners to perform Reiki in the operating room or other hospital settings, was developed by Raven Keyes, a Reiki Master and founder of Medical Reiki™ International. Medical Reiki™ is based on the gold standards and best practices Keyes developed after her 20 years of bringing Reiki into the operating rooms of some of America's top surgeons, including Dr Mehmet Oz and Dr Sheldon Marc Feldman.[30]

Medical Reiki™ training is offered to Reiki Masters in cities throughout the United States. A study that will investigate the use of Reiki in the operating room for women with breast cancer is currently in early developmental stages (Raven Keyes, phone call, February 9, 2020) (see the video: Dr Sheldon Feldman on Reiki and Surgery[31] at https://www.youtube.com/watch?v=X29PZzrgU4I).

Connecting Reiki with Medicine (https://www.reikiwithmedicine.org/), a program under the banner of Full Circle Fund Therapies in the United Kingdom, provides Reiki for hospitalized patients, both children and adults coping with serious illnesses. It is based at the world-renowned teaching hospital and research center St George's in London. The project's goal is to collect data to support Reiki as an evidence-based practice in diverse and acute medical settings. The program provides an in-depth, clinically based training and mentoring program for Reiki practitioners (Feona Gray, phone call, March 19, 2020; email March 20, 2020).

Integrative Medicine Programs

Reiki services are frequently part of integrative medicine programs or clinics. These holistic programs focus on patient-centered care by addressing all aspects of a person's body, mind, and spirit. In 2011, a survey was conducted to determine how integrative medicine was being practiced across the United States. The programs studied offered a variety of services, including medical care, nutritional counseling, acupuncture, meditation, massage, and biofeedback. Fifty-five percent of the clinics used a Reiki or healing touch practitioner either full or part time.[32]

The Integrative Medicine Clinic at Elmhurst Hospital in Illinois opened in 2016 and includes Reiki sessions in its menu of services (https://www.eehealth.org/services/integrative-medicine/. See video: Integrative Medicine at Edward-Elmhurst Health[33] at https://www.youtube.com/watch?time_continue=4&v=XWSvMrXibgA&feature=emb_logo).

Major Health Care Organizations that Offer Reiki Services

Resources for bringing Reiki into health care and community organizations

Nurses are well positioned within administrative and clinical settings to introduce Reiki to colleagues, patients, and families (**Boxes 1** and **2**). The following resources offer information and guidance for nurses interested in establishing Reiki programs in health care or community organizations.

Box 1
Major health care organizations that offer Reiki services

- Brigham and Women's Hospital, Boston Massachusetts
  https://www.brighamandwomens.org/about-bwh/volunteer/reiki-volunteer-program

- Mayo Clinic, Rochester, Minnesota
  https://www.mayoclinic.org/about-mayo-clinic/volunteers/minnesota/service-areas/integrative-healing-enhancement

- Hartford Healthcare, Hartford, Connecticut
  https://hartfordhospital.org/services/integrative-medicine/departments-services/reiki-therapy

- Henry Ford Health System, Detroit, Michigan
  https://www.henryford.com/calendar/wellness/macomb-hospital/healing-therapies-for-cancer-patients

- Cleveland Clinic, Cleveland, Ohio
  https://my.clevelandclinic.org/departments/patient-experience/depts/spiritual-care/healing-services

- Abramson Cancer Center, Philadelphia, Pennsylvania
  https://www.pennmedicine.org/cancer/navigating-cancer-care/treatment-types/integrative-oncology/reiki-therapy

- Dartmouth-Hitchcock Norris Cotton Cancer Center in New Hampshire and Vermont
  https://cancer.dartmouth.edu/patients-families/healing-arts-massage-and-reiki

- Aurora Health Care, Milwaukee, Wisconsin
  https://www.aurorahealthcare.org/services/integrative-medicine/reiki

- Johns Hopkins Integrative Medicine & Digestive Center, Baltimore, Maryland
  https://www.hopkinsmedicine.org/integrative_medicine_digestive_center/services/reiki.html

---

Box 2
Resources for bringing Reiki into health care and community organizations

- Building a Reiki and healing touch volunteer program at an academic medical center[29]
- Development of a hospital Reiki training program, training volunteers to provide Reiki to patients, families, and staff in the acute care setting[24]
- Integrating a Reiki or complementary and alternative medicine program in health care organization; developing a business plan[34]
- Building bridges between conventional and complementary medicine[27]
- Reiki in a cancer center[35]
- Reiki and its journey into a hospital setting[36]
- Providing Reiki in hospitals: practicalities[4]

REIKI FOR SPECIFIC PATIENT POPULATIONS

Reiki's efficacy in the areas of relaxation, pain relief, and alleviation of stress and anxiety[37] potentially makes it clinically appropriate for many types of patient care situations, both inpatient and outpatient. Reiki is easily learned, safe to use, and simply shared with light touch.

Patients with Cancer

People who receive a cancer diagnosis often seek complementary healing modalities to better cope with illnesses that affect the body, mind, emotions, and spirit. Pischke[38] describes the many benefits of providing Reiki to oncology patients in outpatient settings, such as relaxation, pain relief, and a sense of well-being. Reiki research conducted in oncology settings revealed that these patients respond positively to receiving Reiki, showing a lessening of distress, anxiety, depression, and fatigue as well as an improvement in overall quality of life.[39–44] There are also many nonprofit, community-based organizations that offer holistic wellness programs for individuals and families coping with cancer. Wellness House in Hinsdale, Illinois (https://wellnesshouse.org/) is one such example and currently has a long-standing Reiki volunteer and training program for participants.[35]

End-of-Life Care

Reiki has been a part of hospice care since the 1990s.[45] Many hospice programs have trained staff to offer Reiki sessions as part of the care they provide.[46] Terminally ill patients find Reiki beneficial for relaxation, alleviation of pain and discomfort, and relief from anxiety.[47] Reiki treatments are also offered to family members, who often feel helpless as their loved one is dying. Family members who choose to be trained in Reiki can feel empowered and comforted as they share the gentle loving touch of Reiki with loved ones during a sad and challenging time.[45]

Supporting Surgical Patients

The Reiki volunteer program at Portsmouth Regional Hospital in New Hampshire began offering Reiki to presurgical patients in 1997. Positive patient outcomes included increased relaxation and decreased feelings of stress before surgery.[25] Research studies have examined the effects of Reiki on pain in surgical patients. In each study, the treatment groups who received Reiki experienced a decrease in postoperative pain compared with the treatment groups who received sham Reiki and/or no Reiki treatment.[48–51]

Caring for Children

Reiki can be beneficial for children who are seriously ill. Radziewicz and colleagues[52] showed that Reiki therapy can be safely used with no adverse reactions for newborns with neonatal abstinence syndrome in a busy neonatal unit. Two pilot studies have been conducted with children diagnosed with cancer[53] and children receiving palliative care.[54] Both studies provided preliminary evidence for Reiki's effectiveness in managing pain and anxiety with seriously ill children. Kundu and colleagues[55] successfully set up a Reiki training program for caregivers of pediatric medical or oncology inpatients. Participating families reported that Reiki became an effective tool for them to provide comfort, relaxation, and pain relief for their children and helped them feel empowered as active participants in their children's care.

Coping with Depression

A study by Erdogan and Cinar[56] considered elderly residents of a nursing home who were living with depression. The depression scores of the Reiki group were lower than the same scores for the sham-Reiki and no-Reiki groups. Several other studies found Reiki to be helpful for individuals dealing with depression, stress, and anxiety by lessening these symptoms. Those receiving Reiki showed positive effects that lasted over time.[57,58]

Helping Veterans and Others with Posttraumatic Stress Disorder

Studies have been conducted regarding the efficacy of Reiki and other complimentary and integrative health (CIH) modalities in treating veterans, who have a high incidence of pain, anxiety, and depression.[59,60] One of the benefits of many CIH practices is that they offer nonpharmacologic treatment options.[61] The Veterans Health Administration is interested in offering these types of services to veterans.

Reiki has been one of many CIH treatments used specifically for treating posttraumatic stress disorder (PTSD). Reiki services were part of the Fort Hood Texas Reset Program, which treated military personnel for combat-related stress disorders.[62] A study by Church and Brooks[59] reported outcomes for veterans and their spouses participating in a PTSD treatment program that included various complementary therapies, including Reiki. They noted that both veterans and spouses experienced a significant decrease in PTSD symptoms after completing the program.

Many independent Reiki practitioners throughout the United States offer their time and skills to support veterans in the healing process.[63,64]

PTSD is also prevalent in the general population. Experiencing any unexpected extreme stressor can result in ongoing physical and emotional trauma. Examples include natural disasters, physical assault, mass shootings, sexual abuse, serious accidents, or the unexpected loss of a loved one. Police, fire, and emergency service workers tend to have higher rates of PTSD than the general population.[65] Mealer and colleagues[66] found that nurses working in a hospital setting were also susceptible to PTSD.

In her article "Reiki and Post Traumatic Stress Disorder: Healing the Soul," Lipinski[67] presents a detailed discussion about the evolution and symptoms of PTSD and describes how Reiki can contribute to the healing process for any individual with this condition.

Living with Human Immunodeficiency Virus/Acquired Immunodeficiency Syndrome

People who live with acquired immunodeficiency syndrome (AIDS) can benefit from Reiki programs. Schmehr's[68] case study described a person with AIDS who received both Reiki sessions and classes to deal with anxiety, depression, substance abuse, and compliance with his medication protocol. This person reported that adhering to his Reiki self-care program helped him relax, maintain his sobriety, and cope with his depression. His health eventually improved, and he was able to return to part-time work. Several studies describe community programs that have offered Reiki services to people living with human immunodeficiency virus or AIDS and report positive outcomes in terms of pain, stress, anxiety, depression, and insomnia.[69–71]

STATUS OF REIKI RESEARCH

As Reiki is increasingly introduced into health care organizations and more nurses become Reiki practitioners, there is an increased interest and ongoing need for high-quality research that will establish Reiki as an evidence-based practice. Energy-based modalities (EBMs)[12] such as Therapeutic Touch[72] and Healing Touch[73] originated within the nursing profession and have established bodies of research. Reiki training is generic and not specific to nursing practice.[12,13,74] It began as a touch therapy with Eastern origins and was primarily practiced by individuals outside mainstream health care with little empirical evidence of exactly how it worked.[13,74]

Formal Reiki research began in the late 1980s. Over the years, the number of studies has steadily increased. Baldwin[4] reports that, as of June 2019, there are 77 Reiki research articles that have been published in peer-reviewed scientific journals. Systematic reviews of current research report that Reiki shows promise in helping to increase relaxation; reduce pain, anxiety, and depression; and improve general well-being.[37,75] So far, many of these studies have been preliminary, with small sample sizes and study designs that may lack randomization or adequate control groups to address confounding variables.[37] Part of the reason for this is that Reiki investigators have had limited funding and support from research institutions, which subsequently restricts the scope of studies.[75]

To remedy this, investigators have made recommendations for improving design strategies that will better determine the efficacy of Reiki as a complementary therapy in medical care. Some of the major recommendations are:

1. Conduct studies with larger numbers of subjects who have been randomized to treatment and control groups, which will limit the risk of bias and error, and contribute to the overall validity of the study.[37,75–78]
2. Design clinical studies with treatment and control groups that include a Reiki intervention, a sham Reiki intervention, and a nonintervention control group. This type of design potentially controls for the effects of human interaction or attention and the placebo effect.[37,75,76,78,79]
3. Use standardized treatment protocols that include systematic hand placements.[74–76,79] There needs to be better consistency within and across clinical studies for Reiki hand placements to determine whether certain positions are more clinically useful or effective.
4. Design studies that consider both the length and number of Reiki sessions and the overall duration of the treatment protocol.[76,78,79] It has been hypothesized that the effects of Reiki are cumulative and further research is necessary to study the effectiveness of Reiki treatments over extended periods of time.

5. Develop mixed methodological studies that include both quantitative and qualitative research methods. Several researchers have suggested that randomized clinical trials are not as effective in adequately capturing the subtle effects of a vibrational healing practice such as Reiki. As a holistic practice, Reiki engages in whole-person healing.[12,77,80] Mixed designs may be more effective in capturing the more complex, experiential, and balancing aspects of Reiki.[74,77,78]

The Center for Reiki Research (https://www.centerforreikiresearch.org/) website provides a current list of evidence-based research published in peer-reviewed journals along with summaries of each of these studies. A listing of hospitals, clinics, and hospice programs where Reiki sessions are offered is also provided with a link to a description of services or the program. To gain access to site resources, become a member by filling out a simple form at the above link provided earlier. Membership is free.

IMPLICATIONS FOR NURSING

As Reiki becomes more recognized and even more widely established within the health care environment, more nurses will see firsthand the immensely positive impact this healing modality can have on their personal and professional lives. Most importantly, Reiki is a self-care practice that can be easily incorporated into daily life and can support nurses in becoming more mindful in prioritizing their own health and well-being. In learning and practicing Reiki, nurses gain another tool that supports their active participation in personal self-care. Reiki is a whole-person healing approach that sustains body, mind, and spirit. Nurses can model holistic wellness behaviors for their families and friends as well as for patients and clients to emulate.

Nurses can then take the lead by incorporating Reiki into their professional practices as caregivers, teachers, and innovators. Reiki shared at the bedside or in clinic settings can provide gentle comfort and a release of stress and anxiety for patients and families. Nurses can teach Reiki classes to colleagues, patients, families, and community members, offering participants the opportunity to embrace Reiki as a simple but powerful wellness practice that can positively contribute to both health maintenance and disease prevention. Programs have also been developed specifically for caregivers who are providing care for seriously or chronically ill loved ones.[55,81] By learning Reiki, the caregivers can greatly benefit by offering Reiki both to themselves and to those in their care.

Nurses can develop innovative Reiki programs that are beneficial for patients, families, and staff, such as Reiki volunteer programs in outpatient and inpatient areas,[24,29] Reiki in preoperative/postoperative areas,[25] Reiki in neonatal[52] and other intensive care areas,[24] Reiki in palliative care and hospice programs,[46,47] and community Reiki clinics such as https://www.helenewilliamsreiki.com/reiki-clinic.

In our own 25-plus years of Reiki practice, the authors have organized and participated in a variety of Reiki activities to educate and share the gift of Reiki. Based on our experiences, here are some suggestions:

- Teach Reiki in hospital and hospice settings for nursing staff, other health care providers, volunteers, patients, and families
- Conduct informational presentations with brief Reiki sessions for health care providers in hospitals, patient support groups, colleges and schools of nursing, and other community groups
- Provide complimentary Reiki sessions for hospital staff during both nurse and physician appreciation weeks

- Offer presentations with brief Reiki sessions at community health fairs and nonprofit events; for example, American Cancer Society Relay for Life
- Hold Reiki shares/clinics where students can practice and share Reiki with other practitioners and/or the public

Nurses can also be involved in determining future areas for Reiki research, continue to participate in clinical studies, and even gather basic qualitative data. For example, the Full Circle Fund Therapies Connecting Reiki with Medicine program[44] used a simple visual analog scale (VAS) of 0 to 10 and asked patients to subjectively rate their levels of pain, anxiety, and other symptoms before and after short Reiki sessions. All patients (N = 129) experienced an average decrease by 32% in VAS scores for their reported symptoms. This finding is instructive information that can support the efficacy of Reiki and can be shared with both clients and other providers. The possibilities for raising the profile and credibility of Reiki within health care are numerous.

SUMMARY

Health care has made outstanding advances in technology and treatment of many illnesses and diseases. However, there is a resurgence of interest in body, mind, and spirit practices and treatments indicating that society is identifying unmet needs. There is a yearning and desire for both high-tech and low-tech healing modalities. Nurses recognize these needs and are taking leadership roles in advocating and introducing CIH services within health care and community-based organizations. Reiki is a holistic healing practice that is safe, gentle, and noninvasive. The research evidence supporting the efficacy of Reiki will continue to strengthen over the next decade. Reiki is already being embraced and adopted by the nursing profession to meet the healing needs of themselves, their families, their patients and their families, other caregivers, and staff members.

DISCLOSURE

The authors have nothing to disclose.

REFERENCES

1. Clarke TC, Black LI, Stussman BJ, et al. Trends in the use of complementary health approaches among adults: United States, 2002-2012. Natl Health Stat Report 2015;79:1–16. Available at: https://www.ncbi.nlm.nih.gov/pmc/articles/PMC4573565/pdf/nihms720042.pdf. Accessed March 23, 2020.
2. NCCIH National Center for Complementary and Integrative Health. Complementary, Alternative, or Integrative Health: What's in a name?. 2018. Available at: https://nccih.nih.gov/health/integrative-health. Accessed March 23, 2020.
3. Dyer N, Baldwin A, Rand WL. A Large-Scale Effectiveness Trial of Reiki for Physical and Psychological Health. J Altern Complement Med 2019;25(12):1156–62. Available at: https://www.liebertpub.com/doi/pdfplus/10.1089/acm.2019.0022.
4. Baldwin A. Reiki in clinical practice: a science-based guide. Edinburgh (Scotland): Handspring Publishing; 2020.
5. Sacks B. Reiki goes mainstream: Spiritual touch practice now commonplace in hospitals. The Washington Post 2014. Available at: https://www.washingtonpost.com/national/religion/reiki-goes-mainstream-spiritual-touch-practice-now-commonplace-in-hospitals/2014/05/16/9e92223a-dd37-11e3-a837-8835df6c12c4_story.html. Accessed March 17, 2020.

6. Fenwick M, Hutcheson D. More Hospitals Offering Complementary and Alternative Medicine Services. American Hospital Association. Available at: https://www.aha.org/system/files/presscenter/pressrel/2011/110907-pr-camsurvey.pdf. Accessed March 17, 2020.

7. Brusie C. Nurses Ranked Most Honest Profession 18 Years in a Row. 2020. Available at: https://nurse.org/articles/nursing-ranked-most-honest-profession/. Accessed January 08, 2020.

8. Reinhart RJ. Nurses Continue to Rate Highest in Honesty, Ethics. 2020. Available at: https://news.gallup.com/poll/274673/nurses-continue-rate-highest-honesty-ethics.aspx. Accessed January 8, 2020.

9. Brill C, Kashurba M. Each moment of touch. Nurs Adm Q 2001;25(3):8–14. https://doi.org/10.1097/00006216-200104000-00004. Available at: https://www.vivernaluz.org/index_htm_files/Each%20moment%20of%20touch.pdf.

10. Lipinski K. Reiki and Nursing. Reiki News Magazine 2012;11(2):51–5. Available at: https://kathielipinski.com/wp-content/uploads/2018/10/ReikiAndNursing_1_.pdf. Accessed March 17, 2020.

11. Lipinski K. Reiki and the Helping Professions: Caring for yourself first. Reiki News Magazine 2006;5(3):27–9. Available at: https://kathielipinski.com/wp-content/uploads/2018/10/Reiki_and_the_Helping_Professions_Part_I.pdf. Accessed March 17, 2020.

12. Frisch N, Howard K, Butcher HK, et al. Holistic nurses' use of energy-based caring modalities. J Holist Nurs 2018;36(3):210–7.

13. Gallob R. Reiki: a supportive therapy in nursing practice and self-care for nurses. J N Y State Nurses Assoc 2003;34(1):9–13, p11.

14. Vitale AT. Nurses' lived experience of Reiki for self-care. Holist Nurs Pract 2009;23(3):129–45. Available at: https://www.uclahealth.org/rehab/workfiles/urban%20zen/nurses_lived_experience_of_reiki.pdf. Accessed February 28, 2020.

15. Cuneo C, Cooper M, Drew C, et al. The Effect of Reiki on Work-Related Stress of the Registered Nurse. J Holist Nurs 2011;29(1):33–43.

16. Deible S, Fioravanti M, Tarantino B, et al. Implementation of an Integrative Coping and Resiliency Program for Nurses. Glob Adv Health Med 2015;4(1):28–33. Available at: https://www.ncbi.nlm.nih.gov/pmc/articles/PMC4311556/pdf/gahmj.2014.057.pdf. Accessed February 28, 2020.

17. Diaz-Rodriguez L, Arroyo-Morales M, Fernandez-de-las-Penas C, et al. Immediate effects of reiki on heart rate variability, cortisol levels, and body temperature in health care professionals with burnout. Biol Res Nurs 2011;13(4):376–82.

18. Brathovode A. Teaching Nurses Reiki Energy Therapy for Self-Care. Int J Hum Caring 2017;21(1):22–5. Available at: https://www.rwjbh.org/documents/nursing/Teaching-Nurses-Reiki-Energy-Therapy-for-Self-Care.pdf. Accessed February 28, 2020.

19. Stone S. Code Lavender: A tool for staff support. Nursing 2018;48(4):15–7, p.15. Available at: https://my.clevelandclinic.org/-/scassets/files/org/locations/hillcrest-hospital/spiritual-services/code-lavender.ashx?la=en. Accessed March 23, 2020.

20. Johnson B. Code Lavender: initiating holistic rapid response at the Cleveland Clinic. Beginnings American Holistic Nurses Association (AHNA) 2014;34(2):10–1.

21. Maizes V, Rakel D, Niemiec C. Integrative medicine and patient-centered care. Explore (NY) 2009;5(5):277–89.

22. Jayadevappa R, Chhatre S. Patient centered care-a conceptual model and review of the state of the art. Open Health Serv Policy J 2011;4:15–25. Available

at: https://benthamopen.com/contents/pdf/TOHSPJ/TOHSPJ-4-15.pdf.   Accessed March 22, 2020.

23. Wolf J, Niederhauser V, Marshburn D, et al. Defining patient experience. Patient Exp J 2014;1(1):7–19. Available at: https://pxjournal.org/cgi/viewcontent.cgi?article=1004&context=journal. Accessed March 20, 2020.

24. Hahn J, Reilly P, Buchanan T. Development of a hospital Reiki training program: training volunteers to provide Reiki to patients, families, and staff in the acute care setting. Dimens Crit Care Nurs 2014;33(1):15–21. Available at: https://pdfs.semanticscholar.org/fb29/c453e7dbcf01d72e17f3e18b316e2a489c2c.pdf. Accessed March 24, 2020.

25. Alandydy P, Alandydy K. Using Reiki to support surgical patients. J Nurs Care Qual 1999;13(4):89–91.

26. Miles P. Reiki at Portsmouth Regional Hospital. Reiki News Magazine 2004;3(1):26–32.

27. Hartford Hospital Department of Integrative Medicine. Building Bridges between Conventional and Complementary Medicine 2013. Available at: https://hartfordhospital.org/File%20Library/Unassigned/BuildingBridges.pdf. Accessed March 24, 2020.

28. Moore A. Reiki energy medicine; enhancing the healing process. Available at: https://equilibrium-e3.com/images/PDF/ReikiEnergyMedicine.pdf.   Accessed March 24, 2020.

29. Anderson DM, Loth AR, Stuart-Mullen LG, et al. Building a Reiki and Healing Touch volunteer program at an academic medical center. Adv Integr Med 2017;4(2):74–9.

30. What is Medical Reiki?. Available at: https://www.ravenkeyesmedicalreiki.com/ 2017. Accessed March 24, 2020.

31. Dr. Sheldon Feldman on Reiki and Surgery (Video). 2013. Available at: https://www.youtube.com/watch?v=X29PZzrgU4I. Accessed March 24, 2020.

32. Horrigan B, Lewis S, Abrams D, et al. Integrative medicine in America—how integrative medicine is being practiced in clinical centers across the United States. Glob Adv Health Med 2012;1(3):18–94. Available at: https://www.ncbi.nlm.nih.gov/pmc/articles/PMC3833660/pdf/gahmj.2012.1.3.006.pdf. Accessed March 24, 2020.

33. Integrative Medicine at Edward-Elmhurst Health (Video). 2017. Available at: https://www.youtube.com/watch?time_continue=4&v=XWSvMrXibgA&feature=emb_logo. November 8. Accessed March 24, 2020.

34. Vitale A. Initiating a Reiki or CAM Program in a Healthcare Organization-Developing a Business Plan. Holist Nurs Pract 2014;28(6):376–80.

35. Van De Velde J. Reiki in a cancer center. Reiki News Magazine 2012;11(1):27–31.

36. Kryak E, Vitale A. Reiki and Its Journey Into a Hospital Setting. Holist Nurs Pract 2011;25(5):238–45.

37. Baldwin AL, Thompson A. Reiki research: it's time to shift gears. Reiki News Magazine 2019;18(4):19–21. Available at: https://www.centerforreikiresearch.org/timetoshiftgears.aspx. Accessed March 24, 2020.

38. Pischke K. Holistic nursing: integrating Reiki in the oncology setting. Beginnings American Holistic Nurses Association (AHNA) 2018;3:6–7, 20-24. Available at: https://www.apre.pt/ficheirosreiki/3.pdf. Accessed March 23, 2020.

39. Olson K, Hanson J, Michaud M. A phase II trial for the management of pain in advanced cancer patients. J Pain Symptom Manage 2003;26(5):990–7.

40. Fleisher KA, Mackenzie ER, Frankel ES, et al. Integrative Reiki for cancer patients: a program evaluation. Integr Cancer Ther 2014;13(1):62–7.
41. Alarcão Z, Fonseca JRS. The effect of Reiki therapy on quality of life of patients with blood cancer: results from a randomized controlled trial. Eur J Integr Med 2016;8:239–49. Available at: https://www.longdom.org/conference-abstracts-files/2161-0665.C1.025-004.pdf. Accessed March 24, 2020.
42. Chirico A, D'Aiuto G, Penon A, et al. Self-efficacy for coping with cancer enhances the effect of Reiki treatments during the pre-surgery phase of breast cancer patients. Anticancer Res 2017;37(7):3657–65.
43. Potter PJ. Energy therapies in advanced practice oncology: an evidence-informed practice approach. J Adv Pract Oncol 2013;4(3):139–51. Available at: https://www.ncbi.nlm.nih.gov/pubmed/25031994. Accessed March 23, 2020.
44. Martin R, Glanville M, Ball C, et al. Quality Improvement project (QIP) exploring effectiveness of Reiki Therapy on Quality of Life (QoL) outcome measure for Cancer Patients when used in Integrated healthcare (IH). Eur J Surg Oncol 2019;45(11):2228.
45. Barnett L, Babb M, Davidson S. Reiki energy medicine: bringing healing touch into home, hospital and hospice. Rochester (VT): Healing Arts Press; 1996.
46. Forbes N. Reiki trained nurses: integrating energy therapy into palliative care for patients, carers and staff. BMJ Support Palliat Care 2018;8(Suppl_2):A60.
47. Conner K, Anandarajah G. Reiki for hospice patients and their caregivers: an in-depth qualitative study of experiences and effects on symptoms. J Pain Symptom Manage 2017;53(2):420–1.
48. Vitale A, O'Connor P. The effect of Reiki on pain and anxiety in women with abdominal hysterectomies: a quasiexperimental pilot study. Holist Nurs Pract 2006;20(6):263–72.
49. Midilli TS, Gunduzoglu NC. Effects of Reiki on pain and vital signs when applied to the incision area of the body after Caesarean section surgery. Holist Nurs Pract 2016;30(6):368–78.
50. Baldwin AL, Vitale A, Brownell E, et al. Effects of Reiki on pain, anxiety, and blood pressure in patients undergoing knee replacement: a pilot study. Holist Nurs Pract 2017;31(2):80–9.
51. Notte B, Fazzini C, Mooney R. Reiki's effect on patient with total knee arthroplasty: a pilot study. Nursing 2016;46(2):17–23.
52. Radziewicz RM, Wright-Esber S, Zupancic J, et al. Safety of Reiki Therapy for Newborns at Risk for Neonatal Abstinence Syndrome. Holist Nurs Pract 2018;32(2):63–70. Available at: https://www.ncbi.nlm.nih.gov/pmc/articles/PMC5815638/pdf/honup-32-63.pdf.
53. Zucchetti G, Candela F, Bottigelli C, et al. The power of Reiki: feasibility and efficacy of reducing pain in children with cancer undergoing hematopoietic stem cell transplantation. J Pediatr Oncol Nurs 2019;36(5):361–8.
54. Thrane SE, Scott H, Maurer SH, et al. Reiki therapy for symptom management in children receiving palliative care: a pilot study. Am J Hosp Palliat Med 2017;34(4):373–9.
55. Kundu A, Dolan-Oves R, Dimmers M, et al. Reiki training for caregivers of hospitalized pediatric patients: A pilot program. Complement Ther Clin Pract 2013;19(1):50–4. Available at: https://www.ncbi.nlm.nih.gov/pmc/articles/PMC3712613/pdf/nihms-410691.pdf. Accessed March 8, 2020.
56. Erdogan Z, Cinar S. The effect of Reiki on depression in elderly people living in nursing home. Indian J Tradit Know 2016;15(1):35–40.

57. Dressin LJ, Singg S. Effects of Reiki on pain and selected affective and personality variables of chronically ill patients. Subtle Energies and Energy Medicine 1998;9(1):53–82.

58. Shore AG. Long term effects of energetic healing on symptoms of psychological depression and self-perceived stress. Altern Ther Health Med 2004;10(3):42–8.

59. Church D, Brooks AJ. CAM and energy psychology techniques remediate PTSD symptoms in veterans and spouses. Explore (NY) 2014;10(1):24–33.

60. Taylor SL, Hoggatt KJ, Kligler B. Complementary and integrated health approaches: what do veterans use and want? J Gen Intern Med 2019;34:1192–9.

61. Gantt M, Orina JA. Educate, try, and share: a feasibility study to assess the acceptance and use of Reiki as an adjunct therapy for chronic pain in military health care facilities. Mil Med 2019. https://doi.org/10.1093/milmed/usz271.

62. Libretto S, Hilton L, Gordon S, et al. Effects of integrative PTSD treatment in a military health setting. Energy Psychol 2015;7(2):33–44. Available at: https://www.stress.org/wp-content/uploads/2014/02/Integrative-PTSD-Treatment.pdf. Accessed March 15, 2020.

63. Dey E, Emanuel M. Reiki for veterans. Reiki News Magazine 2008;7(4):41–3.

64. Dey E. Reiki resources for veterans. Reiki News Magazine 2010;9(3):61–3.

65. Javidi H, Yadollahie M. Post-traumatic stress disorder. Int J Occup Environ Med 2012;3:2–9. Available at: https://www.theijoem.com/ijoem/index.php/ijoem/article/view/127/247. Accessed March 23, 2020.

66. Mealer M, Burnham EL, Goode CJ, et al. The prevalence and impact of post-traumatic stress disorder and burnout syndrome in nurses. Depress Anxiety 2009;26(12):1118–26. Available at: https://www.ncbi.nlm.nih.gov/pmc/articles/PMC2919801/pdf/nihms211783.pdf. Accessed March 20, 2020.

67. Lipinski K. Reiki and Post Traumatic Stress Disorder: Healing the Soul. Reiki News Magazine 2012;11(4):61–7. Available at: https://kathielipinski.com/wp-content/uploads/2018/10/ReikiAndPTSD.pdf. Accessed March 26, 2020.

68. Schmehr R. Enhancing the treatment of HIV/AIDS with Reiki training and treatment. Altern Ther Health Med 2003;9(2):120, 118.

69. Miles P. Preliminary report on the use of Reiki for HIV-related pain and anxiety. Altern Ther Health Med 2003;9(2):36.

70. Mehl-Madrona L, Renfrew NM, Mainguy B. Qualitative assessment of the impact of implementing Reiki training in a supported residence for people older than 50 years with HIV/AIDS. Perm J 2011;15(3):43–50.

71. Bremner M, Blake BJ, Wagner D, et al. Effects of Reiki with music compared to music only among people living with HIV. J Assoc Nurses AIDS Care 2016;27(5):635–47.

72. Krieger D. The therapeutic touch. New York: Prentice Hall Press; 1979.

73. Hover-Kramer D. Healing Touch: a guidebook for practitioners. 2nd edition. Albany (NY): Delmar Thompson Learning; 2002.

74. Vitale A. An integrative review of Reiki touch therapy research. Holist Nurs Pract 2007;21(4):167–79.

75. Singg S. Use of Reiki as a biofield therapy: An adjunct to conventional medical care. Clin Case Rep Rev 2015;1(3):54–60. Available at: https://www.oatext.com/pdf/CCRR-1-121.pdf.

76. Baldwin AL, Vitale A, Brownell E, et al. The Touchstone Process: an ongoing critical evaluation of Reiki in scientific literature. Holist Nurs Pract 2010;24(5):260–76.

77. vanderVaart S, Gijsen VM, de Wildt SN, et al. A systematic review of the therapeutic effects of Reiki. J Altern Complement Med 2009;15(11):1157–69.

78. Herron-Marx S, Price-Knol F, Burden B, et al. A systematic review of the use of Reiki in health care. Alternative and Complementary Therapies 2008;14(1):37–42.
79. Thrane S, Cohen SM. Effect of Reiki therapy on pain and anxiety in adults: an in-depth literature review of randomized trials with effect size calculations. Pain Manag Nurs 2014;15(4):897–908. Available at: https://www.ncbi.nlm.nih.gov/pmc/articles/PMC4147026/pdf/nihms511785.pdf.
80. Verhoef M, Lewith G, Ritenbaugh C, et al. Complementary and alternative medicine whole systems research: beyond identification of inadequacies of the RCT. Complement Ther Med 2005;13(3):206–12.
81. McCracken J. Teaching Reiki to Caregivers: Reiki for Caregivers and Those They Care for. Reiki News Magazine 2008;7(4):35–9.

Reiki
Defining a Healing Practice for Nursing

Kathie Lipinski, MSN, RN[a],*, Jane Van De Velde, DNP, RN[b,1]

KEYWORDS

- Reiki • Self-care • Nursing • Reiki practice • Energy-based healing • Mikao Usui
- Complementary therapy • Reiki training

KEY POINTS

- The practice of Reiki originated in Japan in the early 1920s and is deeply rooted in Japanese culture, philosophy, and spirituality.
- Reiki is a healing and wellness practice that promotes balance and well-being in body, mind, and spirit.
- Reiki is a complementary or integrative modality used in conjunction with, not in place of, conventional medicine.
- A review of studies has found that Reiki seems to be generally safe, shows no harmful effects for recipients, and has no known contraindications.
- Clinical studies support the efficacy of Reiki in stimulating the relaxation response; decreasing pain and discomfort; and alleviating feelings of stress, worry, and anxiety as well as symptoms of depression.

INTRODUCTION

In the current fast-paced and high-tech health care environment, people are seeking a more holistic, caring, and person-centered approach to health care. With their high level of public trust, nurses play an important role in bridging the gap between conventional medicine and complementary or integrative therapies. To do so, it is important that nurses have a strong foundation and knowledge base of the modalities that they use with their patients or clients.

The Reiki natural system of healing, with its hands-on approach and whole-person orientation, is a natural extension of nursing practice. The study of Reiki offers nurses an opportunity to both care for themselves and create an optimal caring and healing environment for their patients and clients.

[a] Private Practice: Healing from the Heart NY; [b] Private Practice: The Reiki Share Project
[1] Present address: P.O. Box 6983, Villa Park, IL 60181.
* Corresponding author. 224 Village Green Drive, Port Jefferson Station, NY 11776.
E-mail address: kathiekaruna95@aol.com

Nurs Clin N Am 55 (2020) 521–536
https://doi.org/10.1016/j.cnur.2020.06.017
0029-6465/20/© 2020 Elsevier Inc. All rights reserved.

When Reiki is taught from the perspective of the biomedical model, which focuses on treatment and outcome, what is often neglected is the focus on self-care and psychological well-being for the practitioner. The natural healing system of Reiki offers whole-person healing of body, mind, and spirit through regular self-Reiki practice and through the wisdom found in the Reiki Principles, which provide guidelines for present-moment living.

This article provides a thorough description and understanding of Reiki practice so that nurses can recognize the value of Reiki for self-care and the positive impact it can have in their professional work settings.

The Art and Practice of Reiki

To describe the hands-on healing system known as Reiki (pronounced RAY-kee), it is important to understand that the art and practice of Reiki has many layers and is deeply rooted in Japanese culture, philosophy, and spirituality. Hawayo Takata, a Japanese American woman living in Hawaii, brought Reiki to the Western world in the mid-1930s, and what were common beliefs and practices in Japan were difficult to explain and not easily understood by the Western mind. As Reiki expanded in the Western world, much of its spirituality, core teachings, and practices were "lost in translation," making what many people currently practice as Reiki different from what the founder Mikao Usui intended. The healing system known as Reiki includes the vibration or energy that Reiki represents, and the methods used to practice it.

Meaning of the Kanji (Japanese Characters)

The word Reiki is derived from 2 Japanese kanji (written characters or pictograms) that, when drawn, represent a word or phrase. Kanji attempt to convey an idea, an understanding, or the concept of a thing.[1] They are not literal translations. How they are drawn, and their interpretation, can change over time and vary with cultural trends.

As seen in **Fig. 1**, the kanji (or Japanese character):

Rei represents the concept of universal or all around us; spiritual; source or origin; creative intelligence; consciousness; cosmos.

Ki represents the concept of vital force or energy.

The combined kanji for the word Reiki can then represent the understanding or concept of a spiritual life force energy available to all.

From an Eastern perspective, it is thought that this universal field, creative intelligence, or vital force animates, surrounds, and permeates all living things. It supports all of life and, although external, is also within us and interconnects all of life. Life force energy, also known as chi, ki, or prana, flows throughout the body via energetic pathways. When the energy flows freely, the person is in a state of health. Disruption, depletion, or blockage in the flow of this energy may lead to physical disease or psychological or emotional symptoms.[2–5]

WHAT IS REIKI?

Simply stated, Reiki is a healing and wellness practice that promotes balance and well-being in body, mind, and spirit. Within the practice are guidelines for psychological well-being, self-care, working with others, and tools for healing and personal development (discussed later in this article). Reiki is spiritual in that it connects people with their innermost selves and creates harmony between the body, mind, and spirit. It is not a religion and holds no religious creed or doctrine. Reiki is a complementary or integrative modality used in conjunction with, not in place of, conventional medicine.

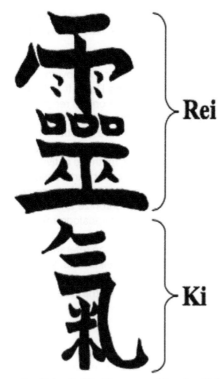

Rei

Ki

Fig. 1. Old-style Japanese kanji for Reiki. (*Courtesy of* Supriya Nair Mumbai, Maharashtra India.)

Reiki has also been described as "a Japanese technique for stress reduction and relaxation that also promotes healing,"[6] "a precise method for connecting universal energy with the body's innate powers of healing,"[7] and "love from the universe, shared through the hands."[8]

At present, the National Center for Complementary and Integrative Health (NCCIH) defines Reiki as "a complementary health approach in which practitioners place their hands lightly on or just above a person, with the goal of directing energy to help facilitate the person's own healing response. It's based on an Eastern belief in an energy that supports the body's innate or natural healing abilities."[9]

Reiki has also been defined as a touch therapy, similar to Therapeutic Touch and Healing Touch, as well as a biofield therapy.[4,10–12]

The term biofield therapies was coined during the US National Institutes of Health (NIH) Conference in 1992[13] to describe noninvasive therapies during which a practitioner works with the subtle vibrational field that surrounds and permeates a person's physical body to stimulate a healing response.[11,13]

The biofield model is based on the principle that all living things are animated with a vital life force that creates a field of energy (biofield) around them. This field is invisible[14] but can be felt and manipulated by a trained practitioner.[10] (see the video: Biofield Science and Healing[15] at https://www.youtube.com/watch?v=vK3YcCn3qSo).

Although almost all of these aspects of the biofield apply to Reiki, what makes Reiki different from other biofield therapies is that the Reiki practitioner simply allows Reiki to flow through their hands to the recipient; there is no manipulation or exchange of energy. The flow of Reiki assists in the restoration of balance on the physical, mental, and emotional levels, so that the recipient's natural ability to heal can be supported and enhanced.[6,7,11]

Most people who offer Reiki quickly begin to recognize that, as the Reiki flows through them, they are connecting with their own loving, compassionate nature and then sharing that with the person receiving Reiki. It is likely that this connection in the practitioner encourages a positive effect on the recipient's experience with Reiki. Studies conducted by the HeartMath Institute on energy exchange between people found that, when humans experience positive emotions such as compassion, gratitude, and caring, the resulting response can be seen in the production of smooth, ordered, and coherent patterns in the heart's rhythmic activity.[16] Researchers also found that the electromagnetic field produced by the heart transmits energy and information between people, and the electrocardiogram signal (measured by the peak of the R wave) from one person's heart could synchronize and be detected in the other person's brain (registered by their electroencephalogram) during physical contact.[16] The researchers were also able to measure the exchange with the subjects placed up to 1.5 m (5 feet) apart.[16] The synchronization referenced in this study could explain what seems to happen during the flow of Reiki. Thus, when Reiki fills a person's bioenergetic field, it is easy to see how it can then spread to others as well as the person's environment (video: Scientific Foundation of the HeartMath System[17] https://www.youtube.com/watch?v=1rstfC0X2ac).

How Does Reiki Work?

Although the mechanism of action for Reiki is currently unknown, Reiki seems to influence the body's autonomic nervous system to move from sympathetic to parasympathetic mode.[18–20] Reiki encourages the relaxation response, and the recipient's natural ability to heal is supported and enhanced.[7] The recipient begins to release tension both physically and mentally. The impact of stress is lessened.

Florence Nightingale, founder of the modern nursing tradition, thought that nature alone cures and described the nurse's role as placing patients in the best condition for nature to act on them.[21] The human body has all the resources and infinitely adaptable systems of checks and balances to self-regulate, repair, regenerate, and thrive. Beginning with the relaxation response, Reiki gently supports the body, mind, and spirit to connect to these natural inner resources in order to heal and return to a state of balance.[7]

Healing Versus Curing

The practice of Reiki places emphasis on healing and not on curing. Western medicine has traditionally focused on disease and the efforts to cure, repair, or modify the course of the disease.[22] In contrast, Reiki focuses on healing, which implies a restoration of balance on all levels of being: body, mind, and spirit. Unlike many Western medical practices, the practice of Reiki is not specific to any disease or illness. Reiki supports the potential for healing by focusing on the individual's innate capacity for renewal and growth on every level of being[7] (see video: What is healing?[23] at https://youtu.be/Kk7kzUt3-Lc).

USES OF REIKI

The list of uses for the healing potential of Reiki is extensive, as shown in **Box 1**.

Reiki is available and accessible to practitioners wherever they go. Because of its simplicity and ease of use, Reiki can be given to oneself or others at home, at work, on a plane, in a car, at school, or just about anywhere. When a friend or loved one

---

Box 1
Uses for the healing potential of Reiki

- Relieves the physical and emotional effects of stress
- Reduces pain and discomfort
- Decreases tension and anxiety
- Improves sleeping patterns and alleviates fatigue
- Prepares and supports a person for surgery, other invasive procedures, and chemotherapy or radiation treatments
- Supports the recovery process from injuries, surgery, or trauma (ie, posttraumatic stress disorder)
- Minimizes or makes more tolerable the side effects of many kinds of treatment or procedures
- Facilitates wound healing
- Supports recovery from addictions
- Supports the resolution of psychological and emotional issues
- Promotes healthy pregnancy and childbirth
- Supports people who are acutely or chronically ill
- Supports caregivers caring for loved ones dealing with acute or chronic illness
- Brings comfort to people who are terminally ill, and can help ease transition
- Enhances personal spiritual development
- Promotes overall health and well-being, and prevention of illness

---

is sad or upset, practitioners can simply place hands on or over the person's back or the heart for emotional support. If someone is in physical pain, practitioners can gently place hands where it hurts. Connecting with Reiki can be done discretely, especially for self-care. For example, if feeling stressed or anxious, practitioners can simply place a hand over the heart or stomach for comfort. When included in family life, Reiki is helpful for childhood ailments, first aid, studying for school, managing the emotions of the teenage years, and so much more. Reiki practitioners who are Reiki master teachers may empower their loved ones to practice Reiki and learn to take care of themselves. Reiki shared in a family or with loved ones is a gift that keeps on giving.

Safety of Reiki

In their review of studies of Reiki, the NCCIH found that Reiki seems to be generally safe and has not shown any harmful effects for recipients.[9,24] There are no known contraindications for Reiki.[24] Because it is simply offered with only a light touch on or slightly above the body, Reiki can be considered noninvasive and nonmanipulative. It is also nonpharmaceutical. Reiki is not a substitute for conventional medical or psychological care. Reiki supports and complements any therapy or treatment a person may be receiving.[24,25] Occasionally, some people experience short-term discomfort after receiving Reiki; it is simply the body releasing stress or toxins as it moves back to a balanced state.

Efficacy of Reiki

Although the large number of reports that describe the many benefits of Reiki have primarily been anecdotal or based on clinical observation, there are clinical studies that support the efficacy of Reiki, in particular with regard to its ability to generate the relaxation response and a decrease of pain and discomfort.[19,26–30] Other studies found that Reiki can alleviate feelings of stress, worry, and anxiety as well as symptoms of depression.[28,31–33]

McManus[34] conducted a review of the literature and concluded that there is reasonably strong evidence for Reiki being more effective than placebo. He also found that Reiki was more effective for decreasing pain, anxiety, and depression and enhancing self-esteem and quality of life for those with chronic health conditions.[34]

The concept of spirituality emerged as a theme in studies by Vitale[35] and Brathovde.[36] Both studies found that nurses who regularly practiced Reiki for self-care reported a deepening of their personal spiritual practices.

Description of a Reiki Session

Reiki can be offered to oneself and others for any amount of time in various settings or situations. Whether in a private practice or a health care setting, it easily adapts to its surroundings and requires no equipment or a special environment. It can be offered as a stand-alone treatment or for support during other procedures. During a Reiki session, recipients are fully clothed and can be in a seated or lying position. Reiki is offered using light touch or hands just above the physical body. The Reiki practitioner can choose to use a more structured approach, going through a series of traditional hand positions that include the areas over the endocrine glands and the major organs that govern the overall body functions. The practitioner may also focus on certain areas of the body and the biofield in response to the recipient's reported physical symptoms and mental-emotional state. Skilled practitioners can also become aware of and treat other areas that seem out of balance as well. Reiki sessions can last from just a few minutes to more than an hour. It is important to be aware of cultural and societal considerations before touching someone. A discussion before the session can be helpful to determine preferences and obtain permission if necessary.

Experience of a Reiki Session

A Reiki session is client focused and varies from session to session. From the practitioner's perspective, Reiki is a neutral, passive practice. During the session, the practitioner is present, supportive, and observant; there is no intent to achieve a certain outcome for the person or attempt to direct the Reiki energy. Recipients receive Reiki in response to their individual needs for healing and balance in the moment. Practitioners cannot give too much Reiki. The wisdom of the body knows how much it needs; when it is returned to balance, Reiki stops flowing.[7]

The response to Reiki varies and it can be a multisensory experience. Recipients may report heat from the practitioner's hands, tingling sensations, or a gentle pulse moving through the body. A sense of peace and slipping into deep sleep is commonly experienced. As the mind quiets, feelings of worry, stress, and anxiety begin to decrease. An emotional release may occur as Reiki gently helps the recipient relax. The effects of Reiki can be subtle and not immediately perceived. Individuals may later experience a night of restful sleep, improved digestion, mental clarity, or a personal insight. The effects of Reiki are cumulative and, with continued practice over time, the personal outcomes can become more meaningful.

Reimbursement and Reiki

Many Reiki practitioners set up private practices in which clients pay for sessions out of pocket. Sessions are usually 30 to 90 minutes in length and rates are comparable with those charged by massage therapists in their area. At present, Reiki is not commonly reimbursed by insurance plans in the United States. However, some insurance companies may cover Reiki when it is woven into a comprehensive treatment plan and delivered by a nurse or a licensed professional.[37,38] Clients can also seek coverage for Reiki services using flexible spending accounts and health savings accounts.

LEARNING REIKI

Reiki is a holistic healing method that can be simply and easily learned by anyone. There are no prerequisites for taking a Reiki class. No particular knowledge or experience is needed to learn Reiki. People of all ages, genders, cultures, and religions practice Reiki. Children often find Reiki appealing and helpful and many are learning how to give Reiki to themselves, their families, and especially their pets.

There are many styles and schools for learning Reiki. Since the early 1930s, the practice of Reiki has continuously evolved and changed, especially with the influence of Western culture. Therefore, a Reiki curriculum is not standardized. Many master teachers vary in their approaches; some teach from a more traditional, Japanese-based perspective. Others teach from an eclectic point of view. Prospective students usually connect with the teacher and style of practice that works best for them. Reiki training is important because it provides people with a form and a structure to work with their own innate abilities to heal.[7]

Some students seek to learn Reiki simply by reading a book or receiving an attunement (a gentle process of empowerment guided by a Reiki master teacher) distantly using the Internet or other streaming services. Reiki is best learned through experience and practice in a live class with a qualified Reiki master teacher who offers guidance, live feedback, immediate answers to questions, and the opportunity to share experience with other students. It is the hands-on attunement from the Reiki master teacher that makes Reiki unique.

Quality Reiki Training

In seeking a competent Reiki teacher, people can start by asking for referrals from friends and families or someone they know who already practices Reiki. People can search the Internet for Reiki teachers nearby. Local health care and community organizations that offer adult education programs often offer Reiki classes. The International Association for Reiki Practitioners (https://iarp.org/) and the International Center for Reiki Training (https://www.reiki.org/) both offer referral services for Reiki master teachers on their websites.

Questions to Ask a Reiki Teacher

When considering a teacher, there are several appropriate questions to ask:

- How many years have you been practicing Reiki?
- Do you practice daily self-treatment?
- What kind of a professional Reiki practice do you have?
- How many years have you been teaching Reiki?
- What style of Reiki do you teach?
- What material do you include in your curriculum and how long are your classes?
- What kind of ongoing support do you offer your students?
- What is the recommended wait time between classes?

CORE COMPONENTS OF REIKI CLASSES

Reiki is an experiential practice and is traditionally taught in 3 or 4 sequential levels.

Dedicated time and practice are encouraged to assimilate the knowledge and master the skills learned at each level. It is generally recommended that students wait a period of time between each class to develop expertise through hands-on experience and practice.

The basic core components included in each class are listed in **Box 2**.

Box 2
Reiki Level I and Reiki Level II

Reiki level I, or First Degree (Shoden)
- Recommended 8 to 10 hours of training
- What Reiki is and how it is used
- Benefits of Reiki
- History of Reiki and the Reiki principles
- Hand positions for offering Reiki to oneself and others
- Reiki level I attunement
- Hands-on practice time offering Reiki to self and others
- Emphasis on self-care and personal practice

Reiki level II, or Second Degree (Okuden)
- Recommended 8 to 10 hours of training
- The Reiki symbols: what they are and how to use them
- Reiki level II attunement
- Hands-on practice time using symbols
- Sending distant Reiki

Auras (energy fields around a person) and chakras (energy centers of the body) are not part of traditional Reiki training but are often included in the curriculum depending on the teacher's training and preference.

A more traditional Japanese style of Reiki class may include elements listed in **Box 3**.

Box 3
Elements of a traditional Japanese style of Reiki class

- Meditation

- Breathing techniques

- Japanese Reiki techniques

- Working with the byosen, the vibration that is emitted from a tense, injured, or ill body part

- Exercises to increase perception in the hands

Reiki Level III or Third Degree (Shinpiden)

After Level II, or Second Degree, there is a wide variety of what the next level is, how students advance, and what is included in class. Reiki Level III, or Third Degree, may be taught as a single class for both master practitioner and teacher. It can also be separated and taught as a Level III class (Advanced or Master Practitioner) and Level IV class (Master Teacher). These classes are often taught in sessions of 3 to 4 days or over a longer period of time and includes various components (**Box 4**).

> **Box 4**
> **Reiki Level III, or Third Degree (Shinpiden)**
>
> - Additional symbols and how to use them
> - Advanced skills and techniques with practice time
> - Ethics, values, and information for setting up private Reiki practice
> - Learning how to perform Reiki attunements
> - Extensive practice time for giving attunements
> - Information and guidance related to organizing and teaching Reiki

Most Reiki Master teachers in the United States issue certificates of attendance or completion to students who attend their classes. Some Reiki programs have requirements that must be completed to receive certificates or move to the advanced practitioner or teacher level. These requirements could include a required number of practice hours or sessions; working with a mentor; coteaching classes; leading a Reiki share or circle where Reiki students, practitioners, and teachers come together to offer Reiki to each other; and offering community presentations. The completion of such requirements is not the equivalent of a formal certification program that has a governing body that provides ongoing assessment of the knowledge and skills required for competent performance in a specific professional role. At present, there are no formalized credentialing or certification programs for Reiki in the United States.

A HISTORY OF REIKI

The history of Reiki is rich but has been cloaked in mystery and misinformation. A more in-depth and accurate accounting of Reiki's history can be found in *This is Reiki* by Frank Arjava Petter,[1] a noted Reiki historian, practitioner, and teacher. New information is being continuously uncovered and shared by others.[6,39–42]

Mikao Usui (1865–1926), founder of the system of Reiki, was born August 15, 1865 in the village of Taniai, in southern Japan. Over the course of his adult life, he was a journalist, a Shinto missionary, an assistant to a prominent Japanese politician, and several other careers that are not known. In his early 50s, he experienced bankruptcy, a situation that led to an identity crisis as he questioned the meaning of his life's work. Usui then began a quest to find his divine purpose and pursued Anjin Ryumei: inner peace or enlightenment.

Usui spent 3 years in retreat at a Kyoto Zen temple (1919–1922) but considered himself no closer to his goal. He then proceeded to the sacred Mount Kurama intending to fast until his death: the final way to attain the state of Anjin Ryumei. After the 20th day, he had a spiritual awakening that led to his enlightenment. He soon realized that he was also gifted with a healing ability when he put his hands on his injured toe and the bleeding stopped immediately.

Usui named his system Shin Shin Kaizen Usui Reiki Ryoho or the Usui Reiki treatment method for improvement of body and mind, to distinguish it from other forms of healing methods already practiced in Japan.[43] He formed the Usui Ryoho Gakkai, an association of Reiki practitioners, and he began to teach and give treatments, spreading Reiki rapidly throughout Japan.

After the death of his teacher Mikao Usui in 1926, Dr Chujiro Hayashi (1880–1940), a retired Naval officer and medical doctor, formed his own association, Hayashi Reiki

Kenkyu Kai (Institute). It was to this clinic that Hawayo Takata, a Japanese American living in Hawaii, came in 1935. After being successfully healed of her many illnesses, Mrs Takata learned Reiki and apprenticed as Dr Hayashi's student. When she returned home to Hawaii, she opened her own practice in Hilo, on the Big Island, and began to give treatments and teach Reiki. In 1938, she invited Dr Hayashi to visit her in Hawaii, where he held 14 seminars and trained 350 students. Thus Mrs Takata and Dr Hayashi began the initial movement of Reiki outside of Japan.[42]

After World War II and the Allied occupation, alternative therapies were banned in Japan and the practice of Reiki was forced to go underground for many years. Very little is known about Mrs Takata's activities after the war until the 1970s, when she began to travel and teach on the US mainland. From 1970 to the time of her death in 1980, she trained 22 or more students as Reiki masters[44] to succeed her and spread Reiki throughout the world.

When Reiki returned to Japan in the late 1980s, it returned as Westernized Reiki, looking much different than the original form. It was not until the late 1990s that information about the original teachings of Mikao Usui and Chujiro Hayashi became more widely known and shared.

Reiki has come full circle, with an increasing interest in learning traditional or Japanese-style Reiki and its historical and cultural roots, thus allowing people to go deeper into the practice with a truer understanding of its spiritual nature and holistic healing benefits.

FOUNDATIONAL ELEMENTS OF REIKI

Throughout the history of Reiki and its ever-evolving styles, certain elements are considered the core of the Reiki system. Although there are variations of the form these elements take, the foundation on which they were built remains the same.[5] These topics are discussed at length in Reiki classes.

Foundational elements of the system of Reiki include:

- The attunement/initiation/empowerment
- The Reiki Principles
- The Reiki symbols
- Treatment
- Personal development

Attunements

The attunement is what sets Reiki apart from other healing modalities and is often clouded in mystique and confusion. Mikao Usui's spiritual awakening on Mt Kurama aligned him with the universal field, vibration, or source of Reiki. His goal then was to help others attain a similar experience and open to their natural healing ability. To help people learn how to use Reiki easily and quickly, Usui developed a process of empowerment that can be referred to as reiju or attunement.

An attunement, in the simplest of terms, is a gentle process of empowerment guided by a Reiki Master teacher. The attunement aligns the person with the vibration of the unlimited source of Reiki. This connection then allows the person to draw on this source. The attunement also balances a person's energy system, bringing the body, mind, and spirit back into harmony.

During an attunement, students sit in a chair with their eyes closed to minimize distractions. Gentle music may play softly in the background to promote a meditative state.

An attunement may sometimes be referred to as initiation: a conscious inner awakening process into a different level of awareness or being.[5] Human beings are all born with a natural ability to heal and bring healing energy to others. The attunement reawakens and reminds the person of this natural ability and alignment with source energy. Once attuned to Reiki, the connection is immediate and lasts a lifetime.

Each degree or level of Reiki includes an attunement. The style and number of attunements per level may vary between lineages/schools.

The Reiki Principles (Also Known as the Reiki Ideals, Reiki Precepts, or Gokai)

Reiki began as a spiritual practice and the Reiki Principles are its heart. Usui designed these principles as guidelines for psychological well-being; he thought that if you healed the mind you healed the body. Usui sensei (teacher) described the principles as "the secret art of inviting happiness… the miraculous cure for all diseases."[6]

The Reiki Principles were originally spoken in Japanese and repeated 3 times because they are considered a kotodama, where the power and spirit of the word come alive when spoken out loud.[1]

The statue that is seen in the video Reiki Principles spoken in Japanese[45] (https://www.youtube.com/watch?v=TlwTyubfXRY) is of Kannon, also known as Kwan Yin, who represents the qualities of mercy and compassion (**Box 5**).

Box 5
The Reiki Principles

Just for today	Kyo dake wa
Do not anger	Ikaruna
Do not worry	Shin pai suna
Be grateful	Kan sha shite
Do your work	Gyo o hageme
Be kind to others	Hito ni shinsetsu ni

Many Reiki practitioners recite them in Japanese every day to honor the original roots of Reiki.

Just for today
The Principles ask that one be mindful and fully present in the moment. When they stay in the moment, they keep their energy and spirit with them instead of sending them out into the future with worries or concerns, or to the past with resentment, blame, or guilt. When focused on the present, one is more aware of the blessings in the present.

Do not anger
Anger keeps one stuck in the past and the past cannot be changed. Attachment to how one thinks people should act and how their lives should be causes pain and suffering. Surrender to what is, trust that everything is exactly as it is supposed to be, and that people and experiences are in one's life to help them grow.

Do not worry
Worry keeps one focused on the future and drains their energy. Let go of worry about what cannot be controlled; attend to what can be. Most things people worry about never happen.

Be grateful
Embracing the "attitude of gratitude" expands and enhances all aspects of life. Being aware of the constant ebb and flow of life and how things can change in a moment reminds people to stay present and savor every moment. Being thankful for people and experiences reminds us how rich our lives really are.

Do your work
Usui Sensei asks one to do what they are meant to do and do it with their whole hearts. People need to live authentically and be true to themselves. Living the compassionate life means that people should live with integrity and follow their beliefs. When people work on themselves, they help heal the world.

Be kind to others
Being kind to others is the golden rule. It is having compassion for all beings, including oneself. It is walking the path of loving kindness, knowing that people are all connected and what affects one affects us all.

The Reiki Symbols

Reiki symbols are an integral part of Reiki practice. Traditionally they have been kept secret and only revealed to students who have reached Second Degree (Level II) and received the corresponding attunement. Part of the secrecy was to respect the tradition and to ensure that students were given all the information and instruction before they began to use them. Nowadays, they are easily found on the Internet.

The Reiki symbols are derived from ancient Sanskrit and Japanese Kanji. They have a form and a mantra (word or phrase) that need to be drawn and/or verbalized to be activated. Usui designed them as tools used as supplements during a Reiki treatment.[42] There are 3 symbols in traditional Usui Reiki: one to work with the physical body, one to work with mental-emotional issues, and one for distant healing. Others have been added over the years as different Reiki systems and styles have been developed. In-depth instructions for how to draw the symbols and what they are used for are given to students in class.

Treatment

Treatment is the foundation of the hands-on practice of Reiki (discussed earlier). Reiki treatment, whether for self or others, touches the physical body and energetically touches the spirit, the mind, and emotions; all levels of a person's being. That is why just a few moments of Reiki can have such a profound effect. Once attuned, people can begin to practice Reiki immediately. Placement of the hands begins Reiki. Removal of the hands stops the flow. It is that simple.[5] No intention is needed. The focus of Reiki is healing for the person's highest good.

As a practitioners give Reiki, it also flows through them and they receive its benefits as well.[7]

Treating oneself is an integral part of the Reiki practice that replenishes the spirit, builds inner resilience, and enhances personal coping skills. A self-care practice can easily be woven into daily life with 5 or 10 minutes throughout the day, in the morning on awakening, or at bedtime (see the video: Self-Reiki: Why you Need this in your Life and how to Do it Effectively[46] at https://youtu.be/niSoR5jFrXg).

Personal Development

Reiki is an invitation for people to open their hearts and live more consciously, bringing more awareness to their everyday lives. People may come to Reiki to learn a relaxation technique to manage stress, but, as they continue to practice, they may begin to move deeper into the spiritual practice. Working with the Reiki Principles on a regular basis teaches people the way of the compassionate heart.

Like a meditation, mindfulness, or yoga practice, Reiki brings people to that quiet place within where they can feel peaceful, calm, grounded, and centered. Accessing that quiet place on a regular basis can bring mental clarity, help develop resiliency,[47] and strengthen the ability to remain calm regardless of the surrounding chaos. With the regular practice of self-Reiki, it becomes easier for people to draw that meditative state into their daily lives. In addition, as they go deeper into their practice, they can better connect to their own inner wisdom to make healthier life choices leading to feelings of personal empowerment.

As people feel more empowered, they grow in self-confidence and self-awareness, feeling more connected to their own personal processes of unfolding and becoming more of who they truly are. A deeper sense of spiritual connectedness, fulfillment, and purpose in life evolves.

SUMMARY

Reiki is a comprehensive holistic healing modality that can be easily learned and incorporated into nurses' personal lives for self-care as well as into their professional lives in caring for their patients or clients. Reiki offers whole-person healing for themselves and others by moving them toward balance and harmony of body, mind, and spirit.

The study of Reiki is often a personal journey and begins as a person searches for a teacher and school or style of practice. Reiki reconnects people to their innate ability to heal; Reiki classes provide the foundation for learning how. As people go deeper into the practice, the Reiki Principles offer guidelines for psychological well-being by reminding people to be mindful: to be fully present in the moment. Reiki self-care practice brings people to a place where they can feel calm, grounded, and centered.

As the profession of nursing continues to grow and evolve, the practice of Reiki can gently return nurses to the foundation of their traditions and knowledge of whole-person healing, and to the art of their practice as providers of compassionate and caring touch-based patient care.

DISCLOSURE

The authors have nothing to disclose.

REFERENCES

1. Petter FA. This is Reiki: transformation of body, mind and soul from the origins to the practice. Twin Lakes (WI): Lotus Press; 2012.
2. Brennan B. Hands of light: a guide to healing through the human energy field. New York: Bantam Books; 1987.
3. Lubeck W, Petter FA, Rand WL. The spirit of Reiki: the complete handbook of the Reiki system. Twin Lakes (WI): Lotus Press; 2001.
4. Rubik B, Muehsam D, Hammerschlag R, et al. Biofield science and healing: history, terminology, and concepts. Glob Adv Health Med 2015;4(Suppl):8–14. Available at: https://www.ncbi.nlm.nih.gov/pmc/articles/PMC4654789/pdf/gahmj.2015.038.suppl.pdf. Accessed January 20, 2020.
5. Pearson N. Foundations of Reiki Ryoho: a manual of Shoden and Okuden. Rochester (VT): Healing Arts Press; 2018.
6. Rand WL. Reiki the healing touch: first and Second degree manual. Southfield (MI): Vision Publication; 2000. p. 3.

7. Barnett L, Babb M, Davidson S. Reiki energy medicine: bringing healing touch into home, hospital and hospice. Rochester (VT): Healing Arts Press; 1996. p. 2.
8. Keyes R. The healing power of Reiki: a modern's master's approach to emotional, spiritual & physical wellness. Woodbury (MN): Llewellyn Publications; 2012. p. 22.
9. NCCIH National Center for Complementary and Integrative Health. Reiki. 2018. Available at: https://nccih.nih.gov/health/reiki-info. Accessed January 10, 2020.
10. Kanherkar R, Stair S, Bhatia-Dey N, et al. Review article: epigenetic mechanisms of integrative medicine. Evid Based Complement Alternat Med 2017;2017. https://doi.org/10.1155/2017/4365429. Available at: https://www.hindawi.com/journals/ecam/2017/4365429/. Accessed January 20, 2020.
11. Dyer N, Baldwin AL, Rand WL. A large-scale effectiveness trial of Reiki for physical and psychological health. J Altern Complement Med 2019;25(12):1156–62. Available at: https://www.liebertpub.com/doi/pdfplus/10.1089/acm.2019.0022.
12. Vitale A. An integrative review of Reiki touch therapy research. Holist Nurs Pract 2007;21(4):167–79. Available at: http://pdfs.semanticscholar.org/05f7/549549378c4d7e2a453c3497e106050678e5.pdf. Accessed February 20, 2020.
13. Jain S, Hammerschlag R, Mills P, et al. Clinical Studies of Biofield Therapies: Summary, Methodological Challenges, and Recommendations. Glob Adv Health Med 2015;4(Suppl):58–66. Available at: https://www.ncbi.nlm.nih.gov/pmc/articles/PMC4654788/. Accessed January 18, 2020.
14. Singg S. Use of Reiki as a biofield therapy: An adjunct to conventional medical care. Clin Case Rep Rev 2015;1(3):54–60. Available at: https://www.oatext.com/pdf/CCRR-1-121.pdf. Accessed February 20, 2020.
15. Biofield Science and Healing (Video). Consciousness and Healing Initiative (CHI). 2017. Available at: https://www.youtube.com/watch?v=vK3YcCn3qSo. July 9. Accessed March 2, 2020.
16. McCraty R. The Energetic heart: Bioelectric Interactions Within and Between People. 2003. Available at: https://www.academia.edu/7289819/The_Energetic_Heart_Bioelectromagnetic_Interactions_Within_and_Between_People. Accessed February 20, 2020.
17. Scientific Foundation of the HeartMath System (Video). 2020. Available at: https://www.youtube.com/watch?v=1rstfC0X2ac. June 18. Accessed February 15, 2020.
18. Baldwin AL, Wagers C, Schwartz GE. Reiki improves heart rate homeostasis in laboratory rats. J Altern Complement Med 2008;14(4):417–22.
19. Diaz-Rodriguez L, Arroyo-Morales M, Fernandez-de-las-Penas C, et al. Immediate effects of reiki on heart rate variability, cortisol levels, and body temperature in health care professionals with burnout. Biol Res Nurs 2011;13(4):376–82.
20. Salles LF, Vannucci L, Siles A, et al. The effect of Reiki on blood hypertension. Acta Paul Enferm 2014;27(5):479–84. Available at: http://www.scielo.br/pdf/ape/v27n5/1982-0194-ape-027-005-0479.pdf. Accessed February 10, 2020.
21. Nightingale F. Notes on Nursing: what it is, and what it is not. Dover Publications; 1969. p. 133.
22. Engebretson J, Wardell DW. Energy based modalities. Nurs Clin North Am 2007;42(2):243–59.
23. What is healing? (Video). 2014. Available at: https://youtube/Kk7kzUt3-Lc. Accessed March 2, 2020.
24. Are there any safety concerns for using Reiki?. Available at: https://www.takingcharge.csh.umn.edu/explore-healing-practices/reiki/are-there-any-safety-concerns-using-reiki. Accessed February 10, 2020.

25. Miles P. Reiki: a comprehensive guide. New York: Penguin Group; 2006.
26. Baldwin AL, Vitale A, Brownell E, et al. Effects of Reiki on Pain, Anxiety, and Blood Pressure in Patients Undergoing Knee Replacement: a Pilot Study. Holist Nurs Pract 2017;31(2):80–9.
27. Olson K, Hanson J, Michaud M. A phase II trial for the management of pain in advanced cancer patients. J Pain Symptom Manage 2003;26(5):990–7.
28. Dressin LJ, Singg S. Effects of Reiki on pain and selected affective and personality variables of chronically ill patients. Subtle Energies and Energy Medicine Journal 1998;9(1):51–82. Available at: http://journals.sfu.ca/seemj/index.php/seemj/article/view/247/210. Accessed February 20, 2020.
29. Notte B, Fazzini C, Mooney R. Reiki's effect on patient with total knee arthroplasty: a pilot study. Nursing 2016;46(2):17–23.
30. Witte D, Dundes L. Harnessing life energy or wishful thinking? Reiki, Placebo Reiki, Meditation and Music. Altern Complement Ther 2001;7(5):304–9.
31. Wardell DW, Engebretson J. Biological correlates of Reiki Touch healing. J Adv Nurs 2001;33(4):439–45.
32. Vitale A, O'Connor P. The effect of Reiki on pain and anxiety in women with abdominal hysterectomies: a quasiexperimental pilot study. Holist Nurs Pract 2006;20(6):263–72. Available at: https://www.academia.edu/28921008/The_effect_of_Reiki_on_pain_and_anxiety_in_women_with_abdominal_hysterectomies_a_quasi-experimental_pilot_study. Accessed February 25, 2020.
33. Shore AG. Long term effects of energetic healing on symptoms of psychological depression and self-perceived stress. Altern Ther Health Med 2004;10(3):42–8.
34. McManus DE. Reiki is better than placebo and has broad potential as a complementary health therapy. J Evid Based Complementary Altern Med 2017;22(4):1051–7. Available at: https://www.ncbi.nlm.nih.gov/pmc/articles/PMC5871310/pdf/10.1177_2156587217728644.pdf. Accessed February 20, 2020.
35. Vitale A. Nurses' Lived Experience of Reiki for Self-Care. Holist Nurs Pract 2009;23(3):129–45. Available at: https://www.uclahealth.org/rehab/workfiles/urban%20zen/nurses_lived_experience_of_reiki.pdf. Accessed March 8, 2020.
36. Brathovde A. Teaching Nurses Reiki Energy Therapy for Self-Care. Int J Hum Caring 2017;21(1):20–5. Available at: https://www.rwjbh.org/documents/nursing/Teaching-Nurses-Reiki-Energy-Therapy-for-Self-Care.pdf. Accessed March 8, 2020.
37. Shepherd-Gentle L. Insurance payments for reiki treatments. International Center for Reiki Training. Available at: https://www.reiki.org/articles/insurance-payments-reiki-treatments. Accessed March 18,2020.
38. Orenstein B. 5 surprising things your health plan may cover. 2016. Available at: https://www.insure.com/health-insurance/what-does-your-health-plan-may-cover.html. Accessed March 18,2020.
39. Fueston R. Reiki: transmissions of light, volume 1: the history and system of Usui Shiki Reiki Ryoho. Twin Lakes (WI): Lotus Press; 2017.
40. Stein J. The Historical Significance of Mikao Usui in Japan. Talk given at Usui Symposium, Berlin, Germany, September 12, 2015. Available at: https://justinstein.academia.edu/research#talks. Accessed February 1, 2020.
41. Stein J. Usui Reiki Ryoho. World Religions and Spirituality. Available at: https://wrldrels.org/2017/01/24/reiki-japan/. Accessed January 10, 2020.
42. Nishina M. Reiki and Japan: a cultural view of western and Japanese Reiki. CreateSpace Independent Publishing Platform; 2017.
43. Rand WL. Reiki before Usui. Available at: https://www.reiki.org/faqs/what-history-reiki. Accessed January 10, 2020.

44. Stein J. Hawayo Takata and the circulatory development of Reiki in the Twentieth century North Pacific [dissertation]. University of Toronto; 2017. Available at: https://tspace.library.utoronto.ca/bitstream/1807/98803/3/Stein_Justin_B_201711_PhD_thesis.pdf. Accessed February 6, 2020.
45. Okazaki M. Gokai - Jikiden Reiki Five Principle in Japanese (Video). 2009. Available at: https://www.youtube.com/watch?v=TlwTyubfXRY. Accessed March 3, 2020.
46. Mainstream Reiki. Self-Reiki: Why you need this in your life and how to do it effectively (Video). 2020. Available at: https://youtube/niSoR5jFrXg. Accessed February 21, 2020.
47. Lipinski K. Reiki, resiliency and self-care. Reiki News Magazine 2015;14(2):35–9. Available at: https://kathielipinski.com/wp-content/uploads/2018/10/Reiki Resiliency_1_.pdf. Accessed February 20, 2020.

Uses of Complementary and Alternative Medicine for Perioperative and Other Patients

Patricia Elizabeth Davies Hall, DNP, APRN, WHNP-BC[a],*,
Elizabeth Borg Card, MSN, APRN, FNP-BC, CPAN, CCRP[b]

KEYWORDS

- Complementary and alternative medicine • Preoperative anxiety
- Postoperative pain

KEY POINTS

- Complementary and Alternative Medicines have been shown to have health benefits for patients experiencing symptoms of anxiety, nausea, pain and have even had efficacious uses for wound healing.
- Complementary and Alternative Medicines are helpful in decreasing post-operative pain in patients who may not be able to tolerate opioids.
- With the opioid epidemic, Complementary and Alternative Medicines may be useful in decreasing the need for as many opioid prescriptions.
- Complementary and Alternative Medicines have potential to help decrease Emergency Department visits for nausea and pain.

BACKGROUND

There are many reasons for pharmaceutical treatments. Health care providers prescribed more than 2.9 billion pharmaceuticals in the office for pain, hypertension, and skin problems and 359 million in emergency departments, mainly for nausea, dizziness, pain, and fluid and electrolyte imbalances.[1] In 2010, 48.3 million procedures and surgeries were performed in the United States.[2] Before surgery, patients may experience anxiety related to the risks, knowledge deficit, and simply the unknown of the experience. After surgical procedures, acute pain and poor tolerance of oral intake are 2 common symptoms patients experience. Not all patients experience the expected healing of a surgical procedure site but, instead, have infections and poor wound healing that often require pharmaceutical treatments.

[a] Belmont University, School of Nursing, 1900 Belmont Boulevard, Nashville, TN 37212, USA;
[b] Nursing Research Office, Vanderbilt University Medical Center, 2611 West End Avenue Suite 328, Nashville, TN 37203, USA
* Corresponding author.
E-mail address: liz.hall@belmont.edu

Nurs Clin N Am 55 (2020) 537–542
https://doi.org/10.1016/j.cnur.2020.06.020
0029-6465/20/© 2020 Elsevier Inc. All rights reserved.

nursing.theclinics.com

Many people desire alternatives to pharmaceutical treatments for various reasons. Some have allergic reactions and others are either unable to afford the cost or choose to not spend money on prescription medication. Parents often choose to not give their children or themselves medications for fear of addiction or other side effects, such as constipation, nausea, and unwanted sedation. An alternative or supplementary pain treatment to opioids, without the accompanying risks would be of value. CAM includes nonpharmaceutical treatments; some examples include acupuncture, essential oils, healing touch, or even certain foods with healing properties, such as honey and ginger.[3] This integrative review of the literature describes some of the applications of CAM within the surgical population. The following databases were searched: Google Scholar, PubMe, and CINHAL. The following key words were used: complementary alternative medicine, postoperative pain, postoperative gastrointestinal distress, therapeutic honey, therapeutic touch, and ginger.

SIGNIFICANCE

Surgical procedures in children and adults present an expected risk of postoperative pain. Postoperative and postanesthesia pain can be intense and difficult to assess with children and even in some adults. Pain assessment of a pediatric postoperative patient easily can be an 8 on the 1 to 10 visual analog scale.[4] Pain has been found to last from the immediate postoperative period to up to 2 weeks later, with the most intense pain reported in the first 12 hours to 36 hours. Typically, between day 3 and day 5, there are significant decreases in pain and a return to normal functioning between day 5 and day 7. A common pattern of postoperative pain is it usually is increased in the morning upon patient awakening and later alleviates due to the administration of analgesics.[4] Many analgesics include narcotics, which have the less than desired side effects of upset stomach producing nausea and vomiting, slowed peristalsis leading to constipation, and sedation posing a risk for injury and decreased respiratory function.[5]

Healing and Comfort

Honey, a natural product of bees, serves to facilitate wound healing and decrease postoperative pain in pediatric patients having certain procedures.[6] Along with honey, essential oils, specifically, peppermint, ginger, and lavender, have been used to promote health benefits for patients experiencing pain and anxiety[7] and nausea.[8,9] Many of these symptoms occur simultaneously before, after, and during surgical procedures in the hospital. Peppermint and lavender combined have shown to alleviate symptoms of headaches,[10] while the linalool, a molecule in the lavender, acts on the limbic system, decreasing feelings of distress, angst, and general anxiety.[7] Inhaled lavender has shown statistically significant in decreasing perceived preoperative anxiety in adult women[7]; aromatherapy massage with lavender is used for preprocedural anxiety in the healing period with burn patients[11] and decreases migraine pain.[12]

Analgesics are a common medication used to manage postsurgical pain in children, and parents often are expected to administer these medications. Parents must be able to recognize when a child is experiencing pain, determine the severity of that pain, and then administer the appropriate amount of analgesics.[13,14] Parents often struggle to manage their child's pain, often using facial grimacing, crying, and lethargy as pain indicators.[4] The lack of guidance, minimal education regarding their child's pain management, and lack of multimodal delivery of expectations contribute to inadequate assessment and management of pain.[13]

Health care providers often desire alternatives when it relates to treatment intervention for children experiencing pain, to complement the effectiveness of the medication. An example of this is use of humor or distraction when administering injectables to children. Nursing protocols using standardized discharge teaching to parents, posed with postoperative pain management for their children, may be useful to increase understanding of safe dosing and improve the patient pain experience.[15]

Unwanted Side Effects

Although opioids and antiemetics are effective means to manage pain and nausea, risk exists of these side effects: respiratory depression, unwanted sedation, nausea, headache, dizziness, somnolence, constipation, and unsteady gait.[5] For any patient needing pain relief, the risk for respiratory depression is of highest priority, among the many side effects caused by opioids. There also is a pervasive fear of addiction among patients that may contribute to the under-administering, thereby increasing discomfort postprocedure. Finally, development of inappropriate chronic pain syndromes, such as hyperalgesia and allodynia, can result after exposure to opioids and poorly managed acute pain.[16] Complementary and alternative medicine (CAM) can meet the need, and the health care culture is acknowledging the potential health benefits for surgical patients during the perioperative period and in the future phases of healing and recovery. The authors' perioperative patient populations have increased awareness and are seeking these alternatives as well. Essential oils are created from plant extracts and offer a tangible way for patients to access and use many CAMs. It is critical to ensure the essential oils used are of the highest quality, with only the plant extracts suspended in unfractionated coconut oil.

Honey

One primary CAM, honey, has been suggested as one method of alleviating throat pain in children postprocedure, specifically tonsillectomy.[17–19] Honey is a natural remedy, with insignificant side effects, that may be useful to reduce opioid usage in postoperative children with throat pain. If less analgesia is required, and acetaminophen or ibuprofen is appropriate to use, the complications and unwanted side effects from opioids then are avoided. Honey has been shown to have relatively inconsequential side effects.[6] Honey does present a risk, however, of botulism in infants. *Clostridium botulinum*, the causative bacteria of botulism, can be present in honey. It generally is recommended that infants less than 1 year of age avoid consuming honey to avoid this complication.[20–22] Adults and children are at risk for poor oral intake after surgical interventions. Honey promotes a faster return to regular oral intake.[23] By expediting the body's tolerance of oral intake, honey counters the risks for constipation, dehydration, and poor healing.

Gastrointestinal Distress and Comfort

Another therapeutic food is ginger, which comes from the plant family Zingiberaceae. There is sufficient evidence that suggests ginger may reduce inflammation and pain.[8] Multipurpose ginger has shown to have health benefits for postoperative patients experiencing pain and inflammation[8,24] and has been shown to decrease the degree of nausea intensity and vomiting symptoms in patients who are pregnant, those receiving treatment of cancer, and those experiencing motion sickness.[8,9,25,26] Ginger also has been used to reduce nausea.[9,24] Alone or combined, peppermint and ginger act to decrease the need for antiemetics postsurgical procedures.[24] Ginger often is ground into powder, turned into a syrup, or extracted as an essential oil.[8]

Acupuncture

Another alternative to using pharmaceutical pain management, which carries risks discussed previously, is acupuncture as a form of therapeutic touch. Acupuncture has been a promising CAM for patients with ongoing pain. Positive outcomes after treatment have been shown statistically significant for patients who have experienced this CAM for pain. Many patients who have undergone a surgical procedure in the past may have chronic low back pain for which evidence supports implementation of acupuncture to improve their perceived quality of life.[27] Additionally, research supports acupuncture as an efficacious intervention for neck pain associated with tension[28] that could prevent a consecutive or future need for a surgical procedure intervention.

NURSING IMPLICATIONS

Patient-centered and holistic nursing care carries the same attributes of altruism as when Florence Nightingale served wounded soldiers during the Crimean war. Watson's caring theory, caritas, of altruism and human understanding, not only is the underpinning of holistic nursing practice but also serves to guide present and future nursing practice.[29] Holistic nursing care embodies each patient as a whole being consisting of a spirit, mind, and body that require different nurturing at different moments of life. The literature reviewed supports the implications of CAM therapy. Nursing care focused on meeting the needs of perioperative patients across the various demographics experiencing pain, anxiety, nausea, and headaches without the high-risk side effects related to opioids and other pharmaceuticals will continue to be implemented holistically. CAM interventions based on the evidence include aromatherapy with essential oils—oral and topical applications that are effective in improving how patients perceive preoperative and postoperative experiences,[5,8,9,24] thus demonstrating self-efficacy in caring for themselves and their children[13,15] and improving postoperative wound healing.[6] When educating patients and their family members, nurses will continue to ensure understanding of instructions prior to patient/parent administration and utilization of CAMs to promote self-efficacy. Providing the best nursing care that current evidence supports to meet individual patient needs is the continued path of nursing as a discipline.

SUMMARY

The efficacy of using CAMs is supported by the literature to decrease preoperative anxiety, postoperative pain and opioid requirements, and nausea and vomiting and to improve severity of headaches and wound healing. Nursing care includes interventions using CAM for treatment of a range of patient needs. Being supportive while educating parents and patients demonstrates altruism, which also is beneficial for improving health outcomes with CAM.

ACKNOWLEDGMENTS

The authors would like to acknowledge the work of Belmont University graduate, Eric Sullivan BSN, RN.

REFERENCES

1. Centers for Disease and Prevention Center, 2013-2016. Available at: https://www. cdc.gov/nchs/fastats/drug-use-therapeutic.htm. Accessed February 14, 2019.
2. Hall MJ, Schwartzman A, Zhang J, et al. Ambulatory surgery data from hospitals and ambulatory surgery centers: United States, 2010. Natl Health Stat Rep 2017;(102):1–15.
3. Available at: https://www.hopkinsmedicine.org/health/wellness-and-prevention/ types-of-complementary-and-alternative-medicine. Accessed February 14, 2019.
4. Gedaly-Duff V, Ziebarth D. Mothers' management of adenoid-tonsillectomy pain in 4 to 8 year-olds: a preliminary study. Pain 1996;57:293–9.
5. Boer H, Forget P. Opioid-related side effects: postoperative ileus, urinary retention, nausea and vomiting, and shivering. A review of the literature. Best Pract Res Clin Anaesthesiol 2017;31(4):499–504.
6. Boroumand P, Zamani MM, Saeed M, et al. Post tonsillectomy pain: can honey reduce the analgesic requirements? Anesth Pain Med 2013;3(1):198–202.
7. Franco L, Blanck TJ, Dugan K, et al. Both lavender fleur oil and unscented oil aromatherapy reduce preoperative anxiety in breast surgery patients: a randomized trial. J Clin Anesth 2016;33:243–9.
8. Singletary K. Ginger: an overview of health benefits. Nutr Today 2010;45(4): 171–83.
9. Ryan JL, Heckler CE, Roscoe JA, et al. Ginger (Zingiber Officinale) reduces acute chemotherapy-induced nausea: a URCC CCOP study of 576 patients. Support Care Cancer 2012;20(7):1479–89.
10. Ahmad R, Naqvi AA, Al-Bukhaytan HM, et al. Evaluation of aromatherapy with lavender oil on academic stress: a randomized placebo controlled clinical trial. Contemp Clin Trials Commun 2019;14:100346.
11. Rafii F, Ameri F, Haghani H, et al. The effect of aromatherapy massage with lavender and chamomile oil on anxiety and sleep quality of patients with burns. Burns 2020;46(1):164–71.
12. Sasannejad P, Saeedi M, Shoeibi A, et al. Lavender essential oil in the treatment of migraine headache: a placebo-controlled clinical trial. Eur Neurol 2012;67(5): 288–91.
13. Nascimento LC, Warnock F, Pan R, et al. Parents' participation in managing their children's postoperative pain at home: an integrative literature review. Pain Manag Nurs 2019;20(5):444–54.
14. Finley GA, McGrath PJ, Forward SP, et al. Parents' management of children's pain following 'minor' surgery. Pain 1996;64:83–7.
15. Jaryszak EM, Lander L, Patel AK, et al. Prolonged recovery after out-patient pediatric adenotonsillectomy. Int J Pediatr Otorhinolaryngol 2011;75(4):585–8.
16. Bell A. The neurobiology of acute pain. Vet J 2018;237:55–62.
17. Hwang SH, Song JN, Jeong YM, et al. The efficacy of honey for ameliorating pain after tonsillectomy: a meta-analysis. Eur Arch Otorhinolaryngol 2016;273:811–8.
18. Lal A, Chohan K, Chohan A, et al. Role of honey after tonsillectomy: a systematic review and meta-analysis of randomized controlled trials. Clin Otolaryngol 2017; 42(3):651–60.
19. Letchumanan P, Rajagopalan R, Kamaruddin MY. Post tonsillectomy pain relief and epithelialization with honey. Turk J Med Sci 2013;43(5):851–7.
20. Wikström S, Holst E. Infant botulism–why honey should be avoided for children up to one year. Lakartidningen 2017;114:ELMF.
21. Long SS. Infant botulism. Pediatr Infect Dis J 2001;20:707–10.

22. Arnon SS. Infant botulism. In: Feigin RD, Cherry JD, editors. Textbook of pediatric infectious disease. 4th edition. Philadelphia: WB Saunders Company; 1998. p. 1570–6.

23. Mohebbi S, Nia HF, Kelantari F, et al. Efficacy of honey in reduction of post tonsillectomy pain, randomized clinical trial. Int J Pediatr Otorhinolaryngol 2014; 78(11):1886–9.

24. Fearrington MA, Qualls BW, Carey MG. Essential oils to reduce postoperative nausea and vomiting. (Report). J Perianesth Nurs 2019;34(5):1047–53.

25. Arslan M, Ozdemir L. Oral intacke of ginger for chemotherapy-induced nausea and vomiting among women with breast cancer. Clin J Oncol Nurs 2015; 19(5):92–7.

26. Bardy J, Slevin NJ, Mais KL, et al. A systematic review of honey uses and its potential value within oncology care. J Clin Nurs 2008;17(19):2604–23.

27. Tousignant-Laflamme Y, Laroche C, Beaulieu C, et al. A randomized trial to determine the duration of analgesia following a 15-and a 30-minute application of acupuncture-like TENS on patients with chronic low back pain. Physiother Theory Pract 2017;33(5):361–9.

28. Araújo W N de, Oliveira L dos SN, Araujo T N de, et al. Effectiveness of acupuncture and myofascial release in analgesia of women with tensional neck pain: Systematic review. Int J Adv Eng Res Sci 2019;6(12). Available at: http://journal-repository.com/index.php/ijaers/article/view/1484.

29. Krol PJ, Lavoie M. From humanism to nihilism: dialectics on Jean Watson's caring theory. Rech Soins Infirm 2015;122:52–66 [in French].

Exercise as a Therapeutic Intervention

Leigh Ann McInnis, PhD, FNP-BC, RN*, Angela Morehead, DNP, FNP-BC, RN

KEYWORDS

- Exercise • Physical activity • Intervention • Therapeutic • Prescription
- Chronic disease • Sedentary

KEY POINTS

- Physical activity recommendations include 150 minutes to 300 minutes a week of moderate-intensity or 75 minutes to 150 minutes a week of vigorous-intensity aerobic activity.
- When compared with no physical activity, engaging in some activity significantly reduces all-cause mortality and reduces cardiovascular mortality.
- Physical activity attenuates age-related endothelial dysfunction, oxidative stress, and chronic inflammation.
- Once medically cleared, providers should use the FITT-VP principle to prescribe exercise for patients.

INTRODUCTION

Noncommunicable diseases (NCDs), such as coronary heart disease, cerebrovascular disease, cancer, diabetes, and mental disorders, are responsible for the majority of deaths worldwide.[1] Physical inactivity and age are primary risk factors for many of these NCDs.[1,2] Sedentary behavior is associated with a 71% increase in mortality, which corresponds with a decrease of 6 years of life. In contrast, individuals who are highly active and nonsedentary have a 32% lower mortality rate, which is associated with an increase of 4 years.[3]

Research shows that any increase in physical activity from baseline makes significant differences in all-cause mortality, cardiovascular mortality, and NCDs.[3–6] Physical activity is considered preventive due to its ability to improve age-related issues, such as arterial and endothelial dysfunction, oxidative stress, and chronic inflammation.[2,7] Evidence also confirms the benefits of exercise as primary and secondary preventative strategies against many chronic diseases.[5] Individuals continue to spend much of their time, however, in sedentary behaviors.[4]

School of Nursing, Middle Tennessee State University, 1500 Greenland Drive, Box 81, Murfreesboro, TN 37132, USA
* Corresponding author.
E-mail address: LeighAnn.McInnis@mtsu.edu

Nurs Clin N Am 55 (2020) 543–556
https://doi.org/10.1016/j.cnur.2020.06.019
0029-6465/20/© 2020 Elsevier Inc. All rights reserved.

Physical inactivity is a modifiable risk factor. Providers are responsible for assessing their patients' levels of activity and explaining the positive effects of exercise and the adverse effects of physical inactivity or sedentary behavior.[8] The beneficial effects of exercise appear to have an inverse dose-related relationship, with all-cause mortality and disease risk decreasing as physical activity increases.[9–11] Regardless of activity level, exercise, as a form of physical activity, should be utilized as an intervention to improve the health and well-being of patients.[8] Discussion of exercise as a therapeutic intervention includes the effects of exercise on the body, the role of medical clearance, and strategies to motivate individuals to increase their physical activity.[12]

PREVALENCE AND IMPACT

Physical activity is an effective intervention strategy for many chronic diseases.[1,5,13–15] Exercise can improve insulin sensitivity, blood pressure, and cognitive function and prevent cardiovascular and cerebrovascular events.[2,16,17] Physical activity provides a 20% to 30% risk reduction for many NCDs.[5] Not only does physical activity have a positive impact on physical health but also it improves mental health, mood, and quality of life.[14,18] In the United States, however, 20% of all deaths are attributed to obesity and physical inactivity.[1] Physical inactivity has been identified as the fourth leading risk factor of global mortality.[1,19] In the United States, 25% of adults sit for more than 8 hours per day.[9] Additionally, leisure-time computer use has increased in all age groups.[20] At the global level, physical inactivity is more common in developed countries, among women, older individuals, and those in lower socioeconomic groups.[9] Physical inactivity and sedentary behavior are known to be independent risk factors for all-cause mortality and many chronic diseases.[16]

In addition to premature mortality and increased morbidity, physical inactivity is responsible for contributing to a significant economic burden.[16] The economic impact includes direct health care costs and losses in productivity.[16] Health care expenditures for patients who report inadequate levels of activity, or activity levels less than guidelines suggest, exceed $90 billion annually. This net expenditure includes costs for all services, including inpatient and outpatient care, home health, and prescription drugs.[21] One health plan reported that if patients increased their activity by 1 day per week, this would decrease health care costs by approximately 4.7% and costs would be cut by 23.5% if activity levels could be increased by 5 days.[21] The prevalence and economic impact of physical inactivity require intervention at the individual and global levels.

RECOMMENDATIONS FOR PHYSICAL ACTIVITY

The second edition of the *Physical Activity Guidelines for Americans* (2018)[6] recommends that to obtain substantial health benefits, adults should engage in at least 150 minutes to 300 minutes a week of moderate-intensity or 75 minutes to 150 minutes a week of vigorous-intensity aerobic activity or a comparable combination. Recommendations regarding muscle-strengthening activities suggest that adults should engage in moderate-intensity or higher-intensity exercise that involves all major muscle groups 2 or more days a week.[6] Benefits of strength training include increased insulin sensitivity, lower blood pressure, and maintenance of strong muscles and bones.[22] Older adults should include exercises for balance training.[6] Older adults and adults with chronic conditions who are able should meet the same recommendations but if not able to do so should engage in as much physical activity as they can to avoid inactivity.[6]

Definitions

When discussing the effects of exercise, the definitions used in the literature must be reviewed. A shared understanding of the terminology provides a foundation for understanding the influence of physical activity on the health of aging individuals and common chronic conditions.

Levels of Physical Activity/Intensity/Exercise

Physical activity is considered any continuous body movement produced by skeletal muscle that increases the use of energy above the resting level.[9] Thus, physical activity includes any type of action, such as walking, jogging, gardening, swimming, or physical labor. This activity can be related to work inside or outside the home, transportation, and leisure time.[8,15]

Exercise is a type of physical activity. Exercise is planned, structured, and repetitive and meant to improve or maintain physical health and fitness.[8] Physical activity is described based on the level of intensity, whether absolute or relative. **Box 1** provides definitions that explain the difference between absolute and relative intensity.[6,23] Another way to evaluate the intensity of physical activity is the talk test.[15] Generally, a person doing a moderate-intensity aerobic exercise can talk, but not sing, during the activity. In contrast, a person doing a vigorous-intensity activity cannot say more than a few words without pausing.[15]

To provide a common language, **Table 1** presents definitions of physical activity intensity, which ranges from light intensity to vigorous intensity, with examples of each intensity level.[6] This differentiation is essential because the recommendations and benefits related to physical activity vary based on the intensity level. **Table 2** presents the terms and definitions describing various physical activity levels.[3,6] These descriptions are necessary because they are used to compare health outcomes throughout the literature. Also, there are several categories of exercise, which include aerobic, muscle strengthening, bone strengthening, balance, flexibility, and high-intensity interval training.[8,15,23] **Table 3** presents definitions of various categories of physical exercise and examples of each.[15] Providers can use these definitions to help guide dosage recommendations for exercise (frequency, intensity, time, and type).[24,25]

PHYSICAL INACTIVITY, AGING, AND EXERCISE

Physical inactivity, obesity, and age influence all body systems and are associated with inflammation and vascular, arterial, and endothelial dysfunction, which are the basis of many NCDs.[1,2,26–29] Exercise is a successful method to prevent many cardiovascular and metabolic disorders, moderate their effects, and even provide

---

Box 1
Absolute versus relative intensity

Absolute intensity is the rate of energy expenditure required to perform any physical activity per minute, without considering cardiorespiratory fitness; it is objectively measured as a metabolic equivalent or MET; The amount of energy expenditure while at rest, for most adults is 1 MET.

Relative intensity uses a person's level of cardiorespiratory fitness to assess the level of effort relative to the individual's fitness using a scale of 0 to 10, where sitting is 0 and the hardest level of effort is 10.

Table 1
Physical activity—intensity

Definitions	Examples
Light-intensity activity: requires <3.0 metabolic equivalent	• Walking at a slow or leisurely activity • Cooking activities • Light household chores
Moderate-intensity activity: requires 3.0–6.0 metabolic equivalent	• Walking briskly (2.5 mph) • Swimming • Tennis (doubles) • General yard work • Bicycling (<10 mph on level terrain) • Active yoga
Vigorous-intensity activity: requires ≥6.0 metabolic equivalent	• Jogging or running • Swimming laps • Tennis (singles) • Heavy yard work (shoveling snow, digging) • Hiking uphill • High-intensity interval training

protective benefits.[1,2,25,27,28] With exercise, skeletal muscle acts as an endocrine organ and stimulates the synthesis and release of peptides, hormone-like factors, and cytokines, which, once combined, are called myokines.[26,27] Through myokines, skeletal muscles can communicate with other organs. Some myokines released with exercise include interleukin (IL)-1β, IL-4, IL-6, IL-15, leukemia inhibitory factor (LIH), irisin, meteorin-like protein (METRNL), follistatin-related protein 1 (FSTL-1), and brain-derived neurotrophic factor (BDNF).[1,29]

ARTERIAL STIFFENING AND NONCOMMUNICABLE DISEASES

The development of vascular dysfunction is connected to many factors, in particular arterial stiffening and endothelial dysfunction.[28] Arterial stiffening, especially of the aorta and carotid arteries, impairs blood flow, which influences endothelial dysfunction, reactive oxygen species (ROS), and inflammation. This vascular impairment is a risk factor for myocardial infarction, cardiovascular disease (CVD), stroke, cognitive decline/dysfunction, hypertension, and chronic kidney disease.[2,26]

Table 2
Levels of physical activity

Term	Definition
Sedentary	Any waking behavior that involves minimal movement or energy expenditure (less than or equal to 1.5 metabolic equivalent)
Inactive	Not getting any moderate or vigorous-intensity physical activity other than movements associated with daily life
Insufficiently active	Achieving some moderate or vigorous-intensity physical activity but less than recommended by physical activity guidelines.
Active	Meeting the physical activity guidelines (150–300 min of moderate-intensity physical activity/wk)
Highly active	Achieving the equivalent of more than 300 min of moderate-intensity physical activity/wk

Table 3
Definitions of types of physical activity/exercise

Activity	Definition	Examples
Aerobic (endurance or cardio activity)	The body's large muscles move rhythmically for a sustained period, causing increased heart and respiratory rate.	Brisk walking Running/jogging Bicycling Swimming Components to consider: intensity, frequency, and duration
Muscle strengthening	Include resistance training and weightlifting These activities increase muscle strength, power, endurance, and mass. Must work all major muscle groups	Using resistance bands Lifting weights Carrying heavy loads Heavy gardening Components to consider: intensity, frequency, sets, and repetitions
Bone strengthening (weight-bearing or weight-loading)	Produce an impact or tension force on the bones promoting bone growth and strength; these activities also can be aerobic and muscle strengthening.	Running Jumping rope Lifting weights
Balance	Improve the ability to resist forces that cause falls. Ability to maintain equilibrium	Walking backward Standing on 1 leg Using a wobble board
Flexibility	Improve the ability of joints to move through a full range of motion	Stretching
High-intensity interval training	Consist of short alternating periods of intense anaerobic exercise with less intense aerobic recovery periods	

In healthy individuals, the large elastic arteries dilate and contract when the left ventricle ejects blood during systole. This elasticity reduces the pressure of blood ejected into the arterial system, decreasing the transmission of high pulse pressures (pulsatility) to organs, such as the kidneys and brain.[27] With age, structural changes to the arterial wall, including degradation of elastin fibers, deposition of collagen, and formation of advanced glycation end products, facilitate arterial stiffening.[2] Oxidative stress and proinflammatory factors also influence arterial stiffness by increasing smooth muscle tone, in part by reducing nitric oxide (NO).[27] With stiffening of the arteries, central blood pressure, peripheral blood pressure, and the work of the heart increase.[23] This increase in blood pressure and change in pulsatility influence the timing of blood flow and decrease perfusion of the heart during diastole.[27] Trauma to the small arterioles and capillaries also occurs as a result of this increased pressure reducing blood flow and oxygen delivery to critical organs. Increased aortic stiffness increases the risk of CVD, cerebrovascular disease, in particular stroke, hypertension, and chronic kidney disease.[27] Aortic stiffness elevates cerebrovascular pulsatility and decreases cerebral blood flow and reactivity and is associated with Alzheimer disease (AD), cognitive decline, and cognitive dysfunction.[2,27]

Exercise improves arterial function, decreases arterial stiffness, and improves elasticity, thereby positively influencing a variety of NCDs. Improved compliance and elasticity of the vessels reduce peripheral and central systolic blood pressure and the overall work of the heart.[2,27] In part, aerobic exercise training moderates the arterial stiffening that occurs with age by increasing the availability of NO. NO, produced by the endothelium, is a potent vasodilator with anticoagulative, antiproliferative, and anti-inflammatory effects.[2,27,28]

Research shows that regularly active individuals and individuals participating in moderate-intensity aerobic exercise have decreased aortic stiffness and increased carotid artery compliance.[2] This decrease in arterial stiffness may be due, in part, to reductions in oxidative stress.[2] Furthermore, Craighead and colleagues[2] report that by decreasing oxidative stress, transforming growth factor β1 is reduced, which decreases collagen and thereby reduces arterial calcification. Anaerobic exercise alone does not produce similar results. If combined with aerobic exercise, results are similar but only when anaerobic exercise occurs before aerobic exercise.[2]

ENDOTHELIAL DYSFUNCTION AND NONCOMMUNICABLE DISEASES

The endothelium plays a critical role in regulating vascular tone, blood flow, metabolism, and immune function.[2,27] With age, however, oxidative stress, characterized by excessive ROS production, contributes to decreased availability of NO and increased endothelial dysfunction.[23] Additionally, reduced antioxidant defenses intensify vascular oxidative stress.[27] Exercise is an essential intervention to combat this age-related deterioration of the endothelium. Exercise facilitates the release of FSTL-1, which promotes overall cardiac health by boosting endothelial function and revascularization of ischemic vessels.[1,29]

Aerobic exercise also stimulates the release of insulinlike growth factor 1 (IGF-1), BDNF, and vascular endothelial growth factor.[17] BDNF and IGF-1 both play a part in the positive effects of exercise on the brain.[17,30] Because IGF-1 is essential for neurogenesis, decreased cognitive function may be due to an age-related decline in IGF-1.[30] BDNF has been associated with metabolism and the formation of new blood vessels, neurons, and memory.[27]

There are many types of cognitive disorders, including AD, vascular dementia, mild cognitive impairment, and Parkinson disease. Researchers agree that physical activity and exercise benefit brain function, memory, academic performance, cognition, decision making, depression, and anxiety.[17,31,32] Myokines also encourage the growth of new synapses and promote the survival of neurons affected by dementia, AD.[31] There also is a growing body of evidence that suggests that exercise interventions enhance and improve the ability of the brain to adapt and respond to changes.[14] This enhancement includes improvement in cognitive function and daily activities. Exercise also lowers levels of inflammation and insulin.[33] Exercise can influence these improvements due to decreased ROS, oxidative stress, and increased blood volume. Additionally, exercise modulates the upregulation of BDNF.[14] Vascular endothelial growth factor increases brain capillary density via the development of new blood vessels. This growth may lead to an improvement in brain perfusion and functioning.[17]

ADIPOSITY, INFLAMMATION, AND NONCOMMUNICABLE DISEASES

Obesity occurs as a result of increased caloric intake and low energy expenditure.[34] As an active endocrine organ, adipose tissue releases free fatty acids, leptin, IL-6, adiponectin, and tumor necrosis factor-alpha (TNF-α), and all can influence other body organs.[34] The distribution of white adipose tissue (WAT), specifically, visceral or abdominal fat, dramatically increases the risk of metabolic disease. WAT also is associated with low fitness, low-grade chronic inflammation, and physical inactivity independent of body mass index.[26,34]

This inactivity starts a cycle of inflammation that initiates the development of visceral fat and promotes inflammation leading to conditions, such as insulin resistance, atherosclerosis, neurodegeneration, tumor growth, and muscle wasting.[1,26,27,29] WAT also is able to secrete proinflammatory cytokines, further exacerbating chronic inflammation.[27] TNF-α and leptin are 2 of the proinflammatory cytokines.[26]

Researchers agree that there is an association between chronic low-level inflammation, CVD, and stroke.[1,27,28] TNF-α is a myokine involved in systemic inflammation, tumor growth, and endothelial dysfunction, which may lead to atherosclerosis. Because TNF-α promotes increased triglycerides, increased low-density lipoprotein, and reduces high-density lipoprotein, it has a significant impact on CVD and all-cause mortality. Some studies show that exercise-induced release of IL-6 inhibits TNF-α.[1] IL-6 plays a central role in reducing the effects of TNF-α by producing anti-inflammatory effects in response to physical exercise, which also decreases tumor growth.[26] Thus, exercise improves arterial and endothelial dysfunction, decreases inflammatory markers, and lowers chronic inflammation, consequently reducing all-cause mortality, cardiovascular mortality, CVD, and strokes.[1,26,27]

Exercise stimulates the release of IL-6, which regulates glucose and lipid metabolism and improves insulin sensitivity.[26] Exercise has been shown to produce a clinically significant improvement in glucose control in patients with type 2 diabetes mellitus. In a randomized study, patients assigned to the experimental group, which added aerobic and anaerobic exercise to standardized treatment, reduction in glucose-lowering medications was seen in 73.5% of patients compared with 26.4% of patients in the control group.[1] Together, IL-6 and IL-15 also have a role in lipolysis, which means they can moderate cholesterol and lipid levels.[26,30] IL-6, working with IL-15, and FSTI-1 have an anti-inflammatory effect that influences long-term improvements on cardiovascular risk factors, including type 2 diabetes mellitus, fat distribution, endothelial function, and the production of acute-phase proteins, such as C-reactive protein.[26,27,30]

In addition to WAT, which stores energy, there is brown adipose tissue (BAT), which burns energy for thermogenesis.[34] Because BAT can burn calories, it has become a new focus for decreasing NCDs through antiobesity and antidiabetic management approaches.[34] Two myokines under investigation due to their role in fat browning are irisin and METRNL. These myokines are activated by exercise and act on adipose and muscle tissue. With elevated irisin levels, there is improved glucose uptake and improved hepatic glucose and lipid metabolism. These effects have a positive impact on hyperlipidemia and hyperglycemia, which often are associated with obesity, metabolic syndrome, and type 2 diabetes mellitus.[35] Irisin and METRNL facilitate insulin sensitivity, thus reducing insulin resistance. Also, irisin and METRNL stimulate, directly and indirectly, the browning of WAT.[34,35] Fat browning is associated with positive effects on obesity-related metabolic problems.[17] Furthermore, irisin is associated with favorable lipid profiles and has an inhibitory effect on adipogenesis. This suggests that irisin may be associated with a decreased risk of NCDs.[35]

EXERCISE AS AN INTERVENTION

There is a considerable amount of research that supports exercise as a first-line treatment of many chronic diseases.[1] The beneficial effects of physical activity are well established, showing reduction of all-cause mortality, CVD stroke, type 2 diabetes mellitus, reduction of cognitive and functional decline, reduced number of falls, and improvement in mental health.[36,37] Individuals with the most mortality benefits are those who have participated in lifelong aerobic physical activity and engage in moderate to vigorous physical activity.[4,28,38] Research shows, however, that the most significant changes in risks are seen by individuals who are inactive or insufficiently active who add physical activity to their routine.[5] This emphasizes the significance of exercise as a therapeutic intervention. Physical activity provides improvements in health and decreased mortality at any age it is introduced.[4,5,28] Many of the health benefits associated with regular physical activity are listed in **Box 2**.[6]

Medical Clearance

Current recommendations from the American College of Sports Medicine include 30 minutes of moderate activity 5 days per week, or 20 minutes of vigorous exercise 3 days per week.[39] It is important, however, to individualize recommendations based on a patient's fitness level and comorbidities.[8] Exercise is safe for most individuals, but there are some risks associated with acute bouts of exercise. The most common risk is musculoskeletal injury, but less common risks include arrhythmia, sudden cardiac death, and myocardial infarction.[40]

To identify patients who are at risk of cardiovascular events, all persons who are planning to start an exercise regimen are encouraged and sometimes required, to

---

Box 2
Health benefits associated with regular physical activity in adults and older adults

Lower risk of all-cause mortality

Lower risk of CVD mortality

Lower risk of CVD (including heart disease and stroke)

Lower risk of hypertension

Lower risk of type 2 diabetes mellitus

Lower risk of adverse blood lipid profile

Lower risk of cancers of the bladder, breast, colon, endometrium, esophagus, kidney, lung, and stomach

Improved cognition

Reduced risk of dementia (including AD)

Improved quality of life

Reduced anxiety

Reduced risk of depression

Improved sleep

Slowed or reduced weight gain

Weight loss, particularly when combined with reduced calorie intake

Prevention of weight regain after initial weight loss

Improved bone health

Improved physical function

Lower risk of falls (older adults)

Lower risk of fall-related injuries (older adults)

have a preparticipation health screening. The screening is done to determine "(a) the current level of physical activity; (b) the presence of known cardiovascular, metabolic, or renal disease (or signs or symptoms of these diseases); and (c) the desired intensity of the exercise bout/program."[39] It is essential for providers who are responsible for patients to evaluate their readiness and ability to exercise. Guidelines include, but are not limited to, the following[8]:

Medical clearance with stress testing recommended

- Patient has current signs and symptoms (chest pain, dyspnea, orthopnea, syncope, murmur, or arrhythmia).
- Patient denies symptoms but has known CVD, diabetes, or kidney disease and has not been participating in moderate-intensity exercise regularly.
- Patient has been participating in moderate-intensity exercise on a regular basis but has not undergone medical clearance in the past 12 months.

Medical clearance not necessary

- Patient denies symptoms but has known CVD, diabetes, or kidney disease and has been participating in moderate-intensity exercise on a regular basis and wishes to continue.[8]

As part of a preparticipation evaluation, it is essential to carefully review medications and their potential to influence physical activity or activity tolerance.[40] Examples of medications that could affect an individual's ability to participate include antihypertensives and statins. Patients on multiple antihypertensive medications may experience orthostatic hypotension, which could cause balance issues and increase risks for falls. Statins also can have harmful effects on physical activity. Most of these are muscular and include myalgia, weakness, muscle cramping, and soreness.[39]

Prescriptions for Exercise

Exploring ways to motivate patients to engage in physical activity is the key to success. Utilization of motivational interviewing and assessing readiness for change may be a part of the process. It is essential that providers who are evaluating patients for readiness and ability to exercise know how to prescribe an exercise regimen appropriately. A prescription for exercise is similar to a prescription for medication; it includes the type of exercise, dose, frequency, duration, and goal.[41] The American College of Sports Medicine agrees and uses the FITT-VP principle to prescribe exercise. A prescription that follows the FITT-VP approach includes frequency, or how often the exercise is done every week; intensity, or how demanding the exercise is; time, or the duration of exercise; type, or the mode of exercise; volume, or the amount of exercise; and progression, or how the exercise advances over time.[42] This template guides the provider to make a specialized program for the patient and takes into consideration not only the patient's ability but also the patient's exercise goals.[42]

When an individualized prescription is written for a patient, Lundqvist and colleagues (2019)[25] noted an increase in physical activity. Additionally, patients who had lower physical activity at baseline had a greater increase in physical activity than those with high levels of physical activity at baseline. Exercise prescriptions have also proved efficacious for increasing functional capacity in patients participating in cardiac rehabilitation[43] and for weight reduction in obese patients who are at risk for osteoarthritis.[44]

Some providers do report barriers to writing a prescription for exercise instead of simply recommending it to patients. Providers self-report low confidence in writing exercise prescriptions, along with acknowledging patients' lack of time and resources.[45]

Another study affirmed that providers perceive that patients have a lack of time or lack of interest and additionally noted that the providers self-report lack knowledge for exercise prescription writing.[46]

Incentives for Exercise

There are different ways to offer incentives for physical activity. Loss-framed incentives are incentives given to individuals and then taken away if a goal is not met. This type of incentive has been demonstrated to be more effective than gain-framed incentives or incentives that are earned only if a goal is met.[47] This information is relevant, especially when encouraging exercise. In 1 study, participants were offered an Apple Watch at a discount with a payment plan option that was dependent on their activity level. Those who had higher activity levels were offered zero or minimal repayment. Loss-framed participants averaged 34% more activity days per month than the gain-framed participants.[47]

Other studies have demonstrated up to a 45% increase in active minutes per week utilizing a short-term incentive that included coffee and movie tickets.[48] Additionally, when financial incentives were offered as a motivator for increased activity, the level of activity has been found to increase as the monetary award amount increased. Identifying motivators is important for companies providing incentives for an activity. Noting this phenomenon will help determine the threshold that motivates participants to increase activity.[49]

One life and health insurance company has initiated programs for its customers to track activity and other healthy behaviors. The participants can earn points and discount coupons that can be used with partners of the company.[50] One company that uses this incentive-based approach reported that it saved more than $4.7 million in medical costs and that there was a 23% increase in its employees' physical activity. Similarly, another insurance company has a plan that offers up to $800 per year to the insured participant if they show proof of attending 12 approved exercise sessions per quarter, and the participants can earn extra incentives by participating in a weight loss program.[51] The participants can earn additional incentives by working with a health coach.[51]

Mobile Applications for Exercise

Exercise applications (apps) are a convenient method of delivery for exercise and physical activity. With more than 77% of adults owning a mobile phone, mobile apps have a far-reaching ability to be utilized by consumers for exercise.[52] Mobile apps for exercise also are cost-effective, and, because they can be customized to individual needs, they are widely accepted.[53] Mobile apps for increasing activity have demonstrated efficacy in multiple populations, including cancer patients[54] and pregnant women.[55] Despite the widespread use of mobile devices in adolescents, this type of delivery of activity information might not be the most efficacious for this population due to the lack of social contact that mobile apps inherently impose.[56]

Mobile apps are successful tools to increase physical activity and improve adherence to exercise regimens. Interactive physical activity apps and step counters also are effective in increasing activity and improving hemoglobin A_{1C} levels in diabetic patients.[53,57] Additionally, a mobile app for activity in patients with a history of myocardial infarction demonstrated increased physical activity along with decreased smoking, increased medication adherence, and overall self-reported improved quality of life in those patients who used the apps.[58] Another study tracking physical activity using a mobile app demonstrated an inverse relationship between daily movement and depression in pregnant women.[59]

Smartphone apps can provide positive effects on physical activity, but the impact differs based on the intervention strategy utilized. Research shows that physical activity is more likely to increase when the duration of use is less than three months. Additionally, improvements in physical activity occur when apps focus on physical activity alone rather than those that combine diet with exercise. However, the research regarding combination apps is limited.[60] These are important factors for providers to consider before recommending an activity app to a patient.

SUMMARY

Prescribing exercise for patients is the best medicine that can be offered. Research shows that exercise is an effective approach to primary and secondary prevention of NCDs. Regardless of when a patient becomes physically active, whether 18 years-old or 80 years-old, exercise significantly decreases morbidity and mortality. Providers must be able to explain the benefits of increasing physical activity to their patients before making recommendations. Understanding the most successful ways to motivate and incentivize patients remains difficult. Sir Howard Stanley, however, explained this best: "Those who think they have no time for bodily exercise will sooner or later have to find time for illness."

DISCLOSURE

The authors have nothing to disclose.

REFERENCES

1. Pedersen BK. The physiology of optimizing health with a focus on exercise as medicine. Annu Rev Physiol 2019;81:607–27.
2. Craighead DH, Freeberg KA, Seals DR. The protective role of regular aerobic exercise on vascular function with aging. Curr Opin Physiol 2019;10:55–63.
3. Bayán-Bravo A, Pérez-Tasigchana RF, López-García E, et al. The association of major patterns of physical activity, sedentary behavior and sleeping with mortality in older adults. J Sports Sci 2019;37(4):424–33.
4. Diaz KM, Duran AT, Colabianchi NC, et al. Potential effects on mortality of replacing sedentary time with short sedentary bouts or physical activity: A national cohort study. Am J Epidemiol 2019;188(3):537–44.
5. Rhodes RE, Janssen I, Bredin SSD, et al. Physical activity: Health impact, prevalence, correlates and interventions. Psychol Health 2017;32(8):942–75.
6. U.S. Department of Health and Human Services. Physical activity guidelines for Americans. 2nd edition. Washington, DC: U.S. Department of Health and Human Services; 2018.
7. Pedersen BK, Saltin B. Exercise as medicine - evidence for prescribing exercise as therapy in 26 different chronic diseases. Scand J Med Sci Sports 2015;(S3):1.
8. Franklin BA, O'Connor FG. Exercise for adults: terminology, patient assessment, and medical clearance. In: Post T, editor. UpToDate. Waltham (MA): UpToDate; 2020. Available at: www.uptodate.com. Accessed February 29, 2020.
9. Peterson DM. The benefits and risks of aerobic exercise. In: Post T, editor. UpToDate. Waltham (MA): UpToDate; 2019. Available at: www.uptodate.com. Accessed February 29, 2020.
10. Missud DC, Parot-Schinkel E, Connan L, et al. Physical activity prescription for general practice patients with cardiovascular risk factors-the PEPPER randomized controlled trial protocol. BMC Public Health 2019;19:688.

11. Shiroma EJ, Lee I, Schepps MA, et al. Physical activity patterns and mortality: The weekend warrior and activity bias. Med Sci Sports Exerc 2019;51(1):35–40.

12. Bachireddy C, Joung A, John LK, et al. Effect of different financial incentive structures on promoting physical activity among adults: a randomized trial. JAMA Netw Open 2019;2(8):e199863.

13. Loprinzi PD, Addoh O. Accelerometer-Determined physical activity and all-cause mortality in a National Prospective cohort study of adults post-acute stroke. Am J Health Promot 2017;32(1):24–7.

14. Cui MY, Lin Y, Sheng JY, et al. Exercise intervention associated with cognitive improvement in Alzheimer's disease. Neural Plast 2018. https://doi.org/10.1155/2018/9234105.

15. Physical Activity Guidelines Advisory Committee. 2018 physical activity guidelines advisory committee scientific report. Washington, DC: U.S. Department of Health and Human Services; 2018.

16. Ding D, Lawson KD, Kolbe-Alexander TL, et al. The economic burden of physical inactivity: a global analysis of major non-communicable diseases. Lancet 2016; 388(10051):1311–24.

17. Kim S, Choi J-Y, Moon S, et al. Roles of myokines in exercise-induced improvement of neuropsychiatric function. Pflugers Arch 2019;(3):491.

18. Del Pozo-Crus B, Carrick-Ranson G, Reading S, et al. The relationship between exercise dose and health-related quality of life with a phase III cardiac rehabilitation program. Qual Life Res 2018;27(4):993–8.

19. Lee DY, Rhee E-J, Cho JH, et al. Appropriate amount of regular exercise is associated with a reduced mortality risk. Med Sci Sports Exerc 2018;50(12):2451–8.

20. Yang L, Cao C, Kantor ED, et al. Trends in sedentary behavior among the US population, 2001-2016. JAMA 2019;321(16):1587–97.

21. Carlson SA, Fulton J, Pratt M, et al. Inadequate physical activity and health care expenditures in the United States. Prog Cardiovasc Dis 2015;57(4):315–23.

22. Hechanova RL, Forest CP, Wegler JL, et al. Exercise: A vitally important prescription. JAAPA 2017;30(4):17–22.

23. Morey MC. Physical activity and exercise in older adults. In: Post T, editor. UpToDate. Waltham (MA): UpToDate; 2019. Available at: www.uptodate.com. Accessed February 29, 2020.

24. Hansen D, Niebauer J, Cornelissen V, et al. Exercise prescription in patients with different combinations of cardiovascular disease risk factors: A consensus statement from the EXPERT working group. Sports Med 2018;48:1781–97.

25. Lundqvist S, Borjesson M, Larsson MEH, et al. Which patients benefit from physical activity on prescription (PAP)? A prospective observational analysis of factors that predict increased physical activity. BMC Public Health 2019;1:1.

26. Ellingsgaard H, Hojman P, Pedersen BK. Exercise and health — emerging roles of IL-6. Curr Opin Physiol 2019;10:49–54.

27. Junior HJC, Gambassi BB, Diniz TA, et al. Inflammatory mechanisms associated with skeletal muscle sequelae after stroke: Role of physical exercise. Mediators Inflamm 2016;1–19. https://doi.org/10.1155/2016/3957958.

28. Rossman MJ, LaRocca TJ, Martens CR, et al. Healthy lifestyle-based approaches for successful vascular aging. J Appl Physiol 2018;125(6):1888–900.

29. Zucker IH, Musch TI. Benefits of exercise training on cardiovascular dysfunction: molecular and integrative. Am J Physiol Heart Circ Physiol 2018;315:H1027–31.

30. Benatti FB, Pedersen BK. Exercise as an anti-inflammatory therapy for rheumatic diseases–myokine regulation. Nat Rev Rheumatol 2015;(2):86.

31. Liu I-T, Lee W-J, Lin S-Y, et al. The therapeutic effects of exercise training on elderly patients with dementia: A randomized controlled trial. Arch Phys Med Rehabil 2020. https://doi.org/10.1016/j.apmr.2020.01.012.
32. Park J, Cohen I. Effects of exercise interventions in older adults with various types of dementia: Systematic review. Activities, Adaptation, & Aging 2019;43(2): 83–117.
33. Bott NT, Bettcher BM, Yokoyama JS, et al. Youthful processing speed in older adults: Genetic, biological, and behavioral predictors of cognitive processing speed trajectories in aging. Front Aging Neurosci 2017. https://doi.org/10.3389/fnagi.2017.00055.
34. Cypess AM, Kahn CR. Brown fat as a therapy for obesity and diabetes. Curr Opin Endocrinol Diabetes Obes 2010;17(2):143–9.
35. Arhire LI, Mihalache L, Covasa M. Irisin: A hope in understanding and managing obesity and metabolic syndrome. Front Endocrinol 2019;10. https://doi.org/10.3389/fendo.2019.00524.
36. de Labra C, Guimaraes-Pinheiro C, Maseda A, et al. Effects of physical exercise interventions in frail older adults: a systematic review of randomized controlled trials. BMC Geriatr 2015;15:1–16.
37. Levinger P, Panisset M, Dunn J, et al. Exercise interveNtion outdoor proJect in the cOmmunitY for older people – the ENJOY Senior Exercise Park project translation research protocol. BMC Public Health 2019;19(1):1–11.
38. Lee PG, Jackson EA, Richardson CR. Exercise prescriptions in older adults. Am Fam Physician 2017;95(7):425–32.
39. Price O, Tsakirides C, Gray M, et al. Pre-participation health screening guidelines. Med Sci Sports Exerc 2019;51(5):1047–54.
40. Zaleski AL, Taylor BA, Panza GA, et al. Coming of age: Considerations in the prescription of exercise for older adults. Methodist DeBakey Cardiovasc J 2016; 12(2):98–104.
41. Seth A. Exercise prescription: what does it mean for primary care? Br J Gen Pract 2014;64(618):12–3.
42. Bushman BA. Developing the P (for Progression) in a FITT-VP Exercise Prescription. ACSMs Health Fit J 2018;22(3):6–9.
43. Gerlach S. Identifying exercise prescription components that predict improvements in functional capacity among participants enrolled in cardiac rehabilitation 2019. Available at: https://digitalrepository.unm.edu/educ_hess_etds/104. Accessed March 3, 2020.
44. Barrow D, Abbate L, Paquette M, et al. Exercise prescription for weight management in obese adults at risk for osteoarthritis: synthesis from a systematic review. BMC Musculoskelet Disord 2019;20(1):1–9.
45. O'Brien MW, Shields CA, Oh P, et al. Effectiveness of the exercise is medicine Canada training workshops on physician counselling and prescription practice: 1084 Board #263. Med Sci Sports Exerc 2017;49:298.
46. Way K, Kannis-Dymand L, Lastella M, et al. Mental health practitioners' reported barriers to prescription of exercise for mental health consumers. Ment Health Phys Act 2018;14:52–60.
47. Hafner M, Pollard J, van Stolk C. Incentives and physical activity: An assessment of the association between Vitality's Active Rewards with Apple Watch benefit and sustained physical activity improvements. Santa Monica (CA): Rand Corporation; 2018.
48. Hajat C, Hasan A, Subel S, et al. The impact of short-term incentives on physical activity in a UK behavioural incentives programme. NPJ Digit Med 2019;2(1):1–6.

49. Rummo PE, Elbel B. Using multiple financial incentive structures to promote sustainable changes in health behaviors. JAMA Netw Open 2019;2(8):e199859.
50. Marr B. This health insurance company tracks customers' exercise and eating habits using big data and Iot. Forbes. 2019. Available at: https://www.forbes.com/sites/bernardmarr/2019/05/27/this-health-insurance-company-tracks-customers-exercise-and-eating-habits-using-big-data-and-iot/#3c04de666ef3. Accessed March 28, 2020.
51. Cigna. Healthy habits incentive instructions 2019. Available at: https://www.cigna.com/iwov-resources/national-second-sale/docs/healthy-benefits/healthy-habits-incentive-instructions.pdf. Accessed March 22, 2020.
52. Mascarenhas MN, Chan JM, Vittinghoff E, et al. Increasing physical activity in mothers using video exercise groups and exercise mobile apps: randomized controlled trial. J Med Internet Res 2018;20:5.
53. Bhattacharyya M. Use of digital mobile apps on exercise may change the behavioural attitude of the south Asian population to improve glycaemic control. Diabetes Prim Care 2019;21:5.
54. Ormel HL, van der Schoot GGF, Westering NL, et al. Self-monitoring physical activity with a smartphone application in cancer patients: a randomized feasibility study (SMART-trial). Support Care Cancer 2018;11(26):3915–23.
55. Choi J, Lee J, Vittinghoff E, et al. mHealth physical activity intervention: a randomized pilot study in physically inactive pregnant women. Matern Child Health J 2016;20(5):1091–101.
56. Depper A, Howe P. Are we fit yet? English adolescent girls' experiences of health and fitness apps. Health Sociol Rev 2017;1(26):98–112.
57. Bentley C, Otesile O, Bacigalupo R, et al. Feasibility study of portable technology for weight loss and HbA1c control in type 2 diabetes. BMC Med Inform Decis Mak 2016;(16):1–15.
58. Johnston N, Bodegard J, Jerström S, et al. Effects of interactive patient smartphone support app on drug adherence and lifestyle changes in myocardial infarction patients: A randomized study. Am Heart J 2016;178:85–94.
59. Faherty L, Hantsoo L, Appleby D, et al. Movement patterns in women at risk for perinatal depression: use of a mood-monitoring mobile application in pregnancy. J Am Med Inform Assoc 2017;4(24):746–53.
60. Romeo A, Edney S, Plotnikoff R, et al. Can smartphone apps increase physical activity? Systematic review and meta-analysis. J Med Internet Res 2019;21:3.

Impact of Therapeutic Music Listening on Intensive Care Unit Patients: A Pilot Study

Stacey G. Browning, DNP, MSN, RN[a],*, Richard Watters, PhD, RN[b],
Clare Thomson-Smith, DNP, JD, RN[c]

KEYWORDS

- Therapeutic music listening • Intensive care unit (ICU) delirium
- Mechanical ventilation

KEY POINTS

- Therapeutic music listening can be applied as a nursing intervention, and it does not require intensive time, financial, or resource allocation, nor does it necessitate members of the health care team learning new skills.
- Delirium can also be described as a manifestation of brain dysfunction that can be present in up to 80% of mechanically ventilated patients in the intensive care unit.
- Mechanical ventilation is an uncomfortable and expensive treatment of patients that can not only increase the risk of developing delirium but also be prolonged with the presence of delirium.
- Patients who develop delirium have longer mechanically ventilated days, increased lengths of stay, and higher rates of morbidity and mortality.

INTRODUCTION

Therapeutic music listening has been used for centuries by various cultures and professions for a wide array of healing and wellness purposes. The Greeks and Romans shared philosophies of therapeutic music listening that included its benefits in healing, increasing or decreasing libido, building charisma, and living in concord.[1] Ancient Chinese used therapeutic music listening to heal the body and mind by providing a harmonious connectedness of the empyreal and Earthly selves.[2] Just as musical styles have evolved throughout history, so too have the uses of therapeutic music listening. At the turn of the twentieth century, music was used to decrease anxiety in patients undergoing terrifying surgical and dental procedures with only local

[a] Whitson-Hester School of Nursing, Tennessee Technological University, P.O. Box 5001, Cookeville, TN 38505, USA; [b] Vanderbilt University School of Nursing, 218 Godchaux Hall, Nashville, TN 37240, USA; [c] Vanderbilt University School of Nursing, 217 Godchaux Hall, Nashville, TN 37240, USA
* Corresponding author.
E-mail addresses: sbrowning@tntech.edu; stacey.browning@mtsu.edu

anesthetic.[3] Music therapy did not become a recognized profession until the conclusion of World War II after professional musicians were used to lift the spirits of soldiers suffering from posttraumatic mental and physical illnesses.[3]

Modern researchers have studied music's effects on patients in many different settings over the last 2 decades.[4] Therapeutic music listening can be applied as a nursing intervention, and it does not require intensive time, financial, or resource allocation nor does it necessitate members of the health care team (HCT) learning new skills.[3–5] Therapeutic music listening refers to passive music listening to prerecorded music. Therapeutic music listening should not be confused with music therapy.[6,7] The American Music Therapy Association, 2020 defines music therapy as, "the clinical and evidence-based use of music interventions to accomplish individualized goals within a therapeutic relationship by a credentialed professional who has completed an approved music therapy program."[6] In other words, music therapists must obtain specific academic degrees and professional certifications/licensure in order to practice in their field of study. An example of music therapy includes a licensed music therapist working with a dementia patient to decrease signs and symptoms of the disease process. Whereas, an example of therapeutic music listening is a patient passively listening to the radio while performing activities of daily living. Comparisons between music therapy and therapeutic music listening as it relates to education and professional requirements are shown in **Table 1**.

Problem of Interest

To date, no studies compare the effects of patient-specific, therapeutic music listening with the incidence and/or duration of delirium among mechanically ventilated (MV)

Table 1
Comparison of music therapy versus therapeutic music listening

	Education & Professional Requirements	Examples
Music Therapy	• Minimum bachelor's degree in music therapy from accredited university 　○ Knowledge in psychology, medicine, and music • Minimum 1200 h of clinical training • Music Therapist-Board Certified (MT-BC) credential 　○ Granted by the Certification Board for Music Therapists (CBMT) 　○ Some states require licensure for board-certified music therapists • Continuing education	• Partnering with patients with neurodegenerative diseases to improve motor function • Partnering with patients of all ages to reduce episodes of pain, asthma, sleep disturbances, etc. • Partnering with patients to lessen symptoms of dementia • Partnering with patients to improve speech, motor skills, and quality of life status after traumatic brain injuries
Therapeutic Music Listening	• None	• Registered Nurses providing patient-specific music listening • Patient listening to music through headphones while participating in physical therapy • Volunteers playing live music or singing to patients in an acute care setting

Data from Definition and Quotes about Music Therapy. musictherapy.org. https://www.musictherapy.org/about/quotes/. Updated 2019. Accessed August 14, 2019.

patients in the intensive care unit (ICU). Results of previous studies support the use of therapeutic music listening in MV patients in various areas of acute care, to reduce physiologic symptoms as well as levels of stress and anxiety.[3–5,7–10] In prior studies, however, patients had to choose their music from a list of selections provided by the researcher, and delirium was not addressed or measured.[4] The current pilot study un-hinged patients from predetermined lists of music, shifting the responsibility of selecting a specific genre or artist, entirely to the patients and their families. As it relates to this pilot study, therapeutic music listening referred to patient-specific, passive listening to prerecorded music that was provided by a registered nurse at timed intervals.

The purpose of this pilot study was to explore the association between therapeutic music listening as a nursing intervention for MV patients in the ICU and the proportion of time the pilot study patients were considered to have delirium, as measured by the Confusion Assessment Method for the ICU (CAM-ICU). Moreover, this study assessed the use of patient-specific choices of therapeutic music listening and the frequency of delirium among MV patients in the ICU.

Literature Synthesis

Delirium is defined as disturbances of consciousness, attention, cognition, and perception that occur over a short period of time (usually hours or days) and fluctuates during the day.[11] Delirium can also be described as a manifestation of brain dysfunction that can be present in up to 80% of MV patients in the ICU.[11] Mechanical ventilation is an uncomfortable and expensive treatment of patients that can not only increase the risk of developing delirium but can also be prolonged with the presence of delirium.[11–13] Mechanical ventilation is the process of bypassing or augmenting spontaneous breathing using a machine called a ventilator whereby breaths are delivered via an endotracheal tube. It contributes upward of $1500 per day to the overall costs associated with receiving care in the ICU. Interventions aimed at reducing mechanical ventilation can significantly decrease total ICU costs.[12,13] Patients who develop delirium have longer MV days, increased lengths of stay (LOS), and higher rates of morbidity and mortality.[11,14–17] Furthermore, delirium in MV patients can lengthen the time spent on a ventilator and increase the risk of death by 3-fold.[11,14,16,17] ICU and total hospital costs associated with delirium in the MV patient population are significantly higher, 39% and 31% (respectively), than costs associated with MV patients who do not experience an episode of delirium.[13] Delirium represents approximately $4 to $16 billion of the annual US health care costs.[18,19]

Although there are no Food and Drug Administration–approved medications to treat delirium, it is often treated with pharmacologic agents.[18,20] The need for an inexpensive and successful intervention is necessary to decrease the incidence of delirium and concurrently morbidity, mortality, LOS in the ICU and hospital, and all costs associated with delirium.[17,19,21] Early recognition of delirium, combined with prompt therapeutic treatment, has potential to improve clinical outcomes by reducing MV days and thereby improving morbidity and mortality, reduce costs associated with complications of delirium, and decrease health care resource consumption.[19]

The presence or absence of delirium among MV patients in an ICU may be assessed with the CAM-ICU, which is paired with the Richmond Agitation-Sedation Scale (RASS) as a 2-part method to determine the constructs of consciousness including the content of consciousness and the level of consciousness, respectively.[10,11,19] The RASS (level of consciousness) score is important to distinguish the CAM-ICU (content of consciousness), because CAM-ICU cannot be performed if the patients' levels of consciousness are too deep to ascertain the content of consciousness.[22] The RASS tool has been validated to distinguish changes in sedation among various critical care patients over consecutive days and has an outstanding interrater reliability (interclass correlation = 0.956; k = 0.73, 95% confidence interval [CI] = 0.71–0.75).[23–25] Nursing staff will perform the RASS first, and if the patient's level of consciousness is greater than or equal to −3, then staff will perform the CAM-ICU. If the RASS is less than −3, the patient's level of consciousness is considered too deeply sedated or unarousable and the CAM-ICU will not be performed. RASS scores are captured as ordinal data with scores ranging from −5 to +4, referenced in **Fig. 1**.

The CAM-ICU assessment has been validated (sensitivity of 93% to 100%; specificity of 98% to 100%; accuracy of 98.4%) with an excellent interrater reliability (k = 0.96, 95% CI = 0.92–0.99) and is the most broadly considered instrument to assess delirium in MV patients in the ICU due to its practicality of use and predictability of morbidity and mortality.[11,19,21,26] The 4 features assessed by CAM-ICU include (1) acute onset of mental status change; (2) inattention; (3) altered level of consciousness; and (4) disorganized thinking as described in **Fig. 2**.[22,26,27] The patient is described as having a positive CAM-ICU (CAM+) if features 1 and 2 and either feature 3 or feature 4 are present.[22,26,27] The CAM-ICU is performed by asking patients a series of questions as well as observing whether patients can follow specific verbal commands (see **Fig. 2**).

Theoretic Framework

To understand the relationship of the entirety of the patients' experiences combined with those of the families and care givers, this study used the person-centered nursing framework, which was developed by McCormack and McCance (2006).[28,29] Person-centered care is a framework that encompasses 4 attributes including *prerequisites*, the *care environment*, *person-centered processes*, and *expected outcomes*[28,29] (**Fig. 3**). *Prerequisites* dictate that nurses should be competent and confident in their clinical knowledge and skills while still maintaining positive interpersonal relationships

Step 1 Level of Consciousness: RASS*

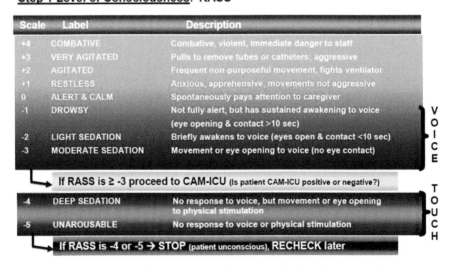

Scale	Label	Description
+4	COMBATIVE	Combative, violent, immediate danger to staff
+3	VERY AGITATED	Pulls to remove tubes or catheters; aggressive
+2	AGITATED	Frequent non-purposeful movement, fights ventilator
+1	RESTLESS	Anxious, apprehensive, movements not aggressive
0	ALERT & CALM	Spontaneously pays attention to caregiver
-1	DROWSY	Not fully alert, but has sustained awakening to voice (eye opening & contact >10 sec)
-2	LIGHT SEDATION	Briefly awakens to voice (eyes open & contact <10 sec)
-3	MODERATE SEDATION	Movement or eye opening to voice (no eye contact)

VOICE

If RASS is ≥ -3 proceed to CAM-ICU (Is patient CAM-ICU positive or negative?)

| -4 | DEEP SEDATION | No response to voice, but movement or eye opening to physical stimulation |
| -5 | UNAROUSABLE | No response to voice or physical stimulation |

TOUCH

If RASS is -4 or -5 → STOP (patient unconscious), **RECHECK later**

Fig. 1. The Richmond Agitation-Sedation Scale. (*From* Ely EW. CAM-ICU Training Manual. Monitoring Delirium in the ICU. icudelirium.org. https://www.icudelirium.org/medical-professionals/delirium/monitoring-delirium-in-the-icu. Published 2002. Updated 2016. Accessed January 25, 2020; with permission.)

Step 2 Content of Consciousness: CAM-ICU

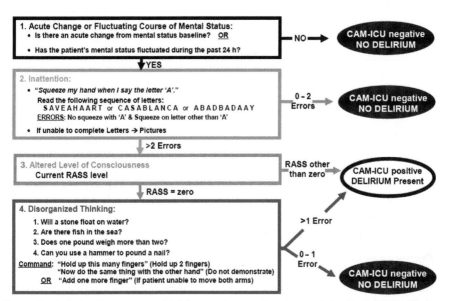

Fig. 2. Confusion Assessment Method for Use in Intensive Care Unit Patients. (*From* Ely EW. CAM-ICU Training Manual. Monitoring Delirium in the ICU. icudelirium.org. https://www. icudelirium.org/medical-professionals/delirium/monitoring-delirium-in-the-icu. Published 2002. Updated 2016. Accessed January 25, 2020; with permission.)

with patients, families, and coworkers that model their values and beliefs.[28,29] The primary investigator (PI) was a former nurse leader in the MICU who had fostered positive professional relationships with nurse and physician leaders, as well as all members of the HCT. The PI provided a presentation to all unit staff before the pilot study in order to encourage collegiality and buy-in from the bedside clinicians.

Collegiality, shared decision-making that is supported by organizational leadership and systems, and innovation are all criteria that contribute to the *care environment*.[28–30] Supportive leaders and a focus on evidence-based practice are fundamental to the success of a person-centered care environment. Operationalizing person-centered nursing highly depends on the care environment. The MICU leadership and clinicians partnered with the PI and encouraged evidence-based processes and supported therapeutic music listening for patients.

Person-centered processes assert health care clinicians should share decision-making with patients and families and cater to their values, beliefs, and needs that will create the best outcomes based on what the patients deem most important.[28–30] Nurse-to-patient engagement is significant to the success of the person-centered process. All patients and their respective families who were recruited to participate in the pilot study were encouraged to share their values, beliefs, and needs in terms of their music selections and desired outcomes. Patient self-determination in health care is an important part of person-centered processes and care, and it is also protected by federal law.[31] Emphasis on limitless music options was important to encourage the rights of the patients and families to choose.

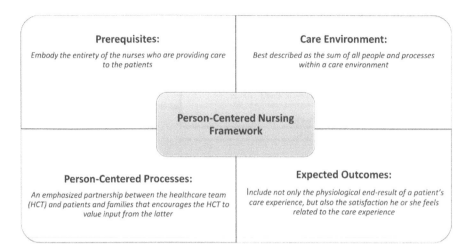

Fig. 3. Person-Centered Nursing Framework. (*Data from* McCormack B, McCance T. Development of a framework for person-centred nursing. Journal of Advanced Nursing 2006;56(5):472-479.)

Outcomes include not only the physiologic end-result of a patient's care experience but also the satisfaction he or she feels related to the care experience.[28–30,32] It is important to be able to measure the outcomes related to person-centered nursing. The measurable outcome of the MUSIC Pilot was the presence or absence, as well as the incidence of delirium among MV patients who received the therapeutic, person-centered nursing intervention consisting of prescribed dosing intervals of patient-specific and self-determined therapeutic music.

METHODS

This pilot study was a prospective cohort design performed in a medical ICU (MICU) at a tertiary, metropolitan medical center. For the duration of this pilot study, the MICU was a 34-bed unit that treated a wide variety of patients, with more than 3000 patients per year being admitted. The top 10 diagnoses of MICU patients were:

1. Other (19.1%)
2. Gastrointestinal bleeding (11%)
3. Sepsis (10.5%)
4. Respiratory failure (7.6%)
5. Altered mental status/coma (4.6%)
6. Shortness of breath/dyspnea (4.6%)
7. Pneumonia/empyema (4.2%)
8. Overdose/intoxication/poisoning (3.7%)
9. Diabetic ketoacidosis/hyperglycemia (3.2%)
10. Surgical complication (2.6%)

The category titled "other" included such diagnoses as organ donation, abscess, failure to thrive, cellulitis, nausea/vomiting, and many others that did not fit into a provided diagnosis list. Considering the different types of diagnoses in the MICU, there was a high frequency of MV patients with a high severity of illness. A higher level of severity of illness contributes to an increased risk of delirium.[17,33]

Recruitment

The inclusion criteria consisted of patients in the MICU who were MV. Exclusion criteria included the following patient populations:

- Hard of hearing or hearing impaired
- Baseline cognitive dysfunction
- Prisoners
- Moribund
- Receiving comfort or end-of-life care
- No family or friends present

Patients were enrolled by the PI following study approval by the medical center's Institutional Review Board. Of the 6 enrolled patients, 3 were randomized to the pilot group and 3 were randomized to the control group using a randomizing table. Sixty-seven percent (n = 2) of the pilot group patients were men, and 33% were women (n = 1). Two were admitted with a primary pulmonary diagnosis and the other was admitted with a medical (nonpulmonary) diagnosis. Primary pulmonary diagnoses included respiratory failure, shortness of breath, dyspnea, pneumonia, and/or empyema. In the control group, all 3 of the patients were women (n = 3; 100%), with 2 admitting diagnoses of pulmonary (67%) and 1 medical (33%) (nonpulmonary) condition (**Table 2**).

The organization's standard of care consisted of nurses assessing and documenting the RASS and CAM-ICU scores for every MV patient every 8 to 12 hours (once per shift) or with any clinical or MV changes. Every MICU bed had the capacity to provide nature sounds, classical music, or light jazz. Every MICU patient room was equipped with a computer or workstation on wheels through which any type of music could be provided by using free streaming applications. Before this pilot study, the audio tools available to the unit staff and patients were used infrequently and at irregular intervals.

Intervention and Procedure

Enrolling participants was accomplished by recruiting MV patients and their family members so that they were all active partners in the pilot study, as well as advocates for their loved ones. The PI and family members interacted with the pilot study patients in order to establish patient-centric music selections. During the study period, therapeutic music listening was provided by the PI at prescribed dosing intervals defined as 1-hour increments, twice daily from 10:00 AM to 11:00 AM and from 9:00 PM until 10:00 PM The music was delivered using free streaming applications on the computers

Table 2
Patient demographic characteristics

	PILOT Group (n = 3)	CONTROL Group (n = 3)
Age		
Mean ± SD (range)	64 ± 12.96 (30)	71 ± 4.51 (10)
Gender		
Female (%)	1 (33%)	3 (100%)
Male (%)	2 (67%)	0 (0%)
Admission diagnosis		
Pulmonary (%)	2 (67%)	2 (67%)
Nonpulmonary (%)	1 (33%)	1 (33%)
Length of stay before enrolment		
Median (range)	9 (21)	3 (5)

located in every patient room. More music listening was provided by the primary bedside nurses if the pilot study patients or families requested it in excess of the prescribed dosing intervals. During the prescribed dosing intervals, the PI performed chart reviews on all the enrolled MV patients in the MICU to obtain their documented RASS and CAM-ICU scores. All RASS and CAM-ICU scores were documented in the electronic medical records for all MV patients in the MICU as part of the organization's standard of care. Standard of care dictates RASS and CAM-ICU assessments are performed and recorded in the patients' charts every 8 to 12 hours (or once per shift) or as needed with any change in clinical or MV status.[34,35] The proportion of time patients were considered CAM+, measured by positive CAM-ICU assessments, was compared between the 2 groups with $n = 3$ for each subsequent group.

Data Analysis

The expected primary outcome was to decrease the proportion of time a patient was scored as CAM+. CAM-ICU scores could have been recorded as either binary, as in the case of recording either CAM+ or CAM−, or continuous if measured as the percent of time the patient was CAM+. For this pilot study, CAM-ICU scores were recorded as the percent of time the patient was CAM+. If the data had been normally distributed, a Student's t-test would have been used to determine the statistical significance. If the data had been abnormally distributed, the Kruskal-Wallace one-way analysis of variance would have been used after the medians, and interquartile ranges were determined for the music and control groups. Conversely, the primary outcome could have also been recorded as the proportion of patients who had never scored CAM+. With the latter method of displaying data, the outcomes would have been binary, and the chi-square test would have determined whether there was statistical significance between the observed and the expected frequencies. If the groups were not equal at baseline, I would have adjusted for the abnormalities in covariates.

RASS scores were captured for each patient as ordinal data with scores ranging from −5 to +4. As a secondary outcome, the mean RASS for each patient group (music vs control) was captured as well as the medians and standard deviations. With a larger sample size and concurrently a larger data set, once plotted, an analysis under the curve would have provided an integrated measurement of RASS.

RESULTS

The purpose of this pilot study was to explore the association between therapeutic music listening as a nursing intervention for MV patients in the ICU and the incidence and duration of delirium among the pilot study patients, as measured by the CAM-ICU. Two metrics were assessed, documented, and evaluated, including the RASS and CAM-ICU scores. Recalling the RASS scale from **Fig. 1**, an RASS score of 0 meant the patient was alert and calm, whereas scores ranging from +1 to +4 indicated the patient was restless, agitated, very agitated, and combative, respectively. RASS scores ranging from −5 to −1 indicated the patient was unarousable, deeply sedated, lightly sedated, or drowsy, respectively. If the patients scored less than −3, the CAM-ICU assessment was not performed, as the patients were deemed unconscious per the RASS scale. This pilot study's mean RASS scores suggested that the MUSIC group ($n = 3$) spent more time alert and calm to agitated (1.3 ± 1.2(5)), whereas the control group ($n = 3$) seemed to fluctuate between sedated (2.7 ± 1.7(4)) and agitated (1 ± 0.8(2)) as noted in **Table 3**.

CAM-ICU scores were measured as continuous as the percentage of time the patients in each group were CAM+, which indicates the presence of ICU delirium.

Table 3
Richmond Agitation-Sedation Scale data

Outcome	MUSIC Group (n = 3)	CONTROL Group (n = 3)
RASS ≥0 mean ± SD (range)	1.3 ± 1.2 (5)	1 ± 0.8 (2)
RASS <0 mean ± SD (range)	3 ± 1 (0)	2.7 ± 1.7 (4)

Patients who received an RASS score greater than or equal to −3 were awake and alert enough to perform the CAM-ICU assessment. Because of the small number of pilot study participants, there was no statistical significance assigned to the data. However, the MUSIC group (n = 3) experienced less proportion of time with documented ICU delirium (33%) than the control group (n = 3) did (67%) (**Fig. 4**).

DISCUSSION

This pilot study examined the relationship between nurse-driven, therapeutic music listening and the proportion of time MV patients in the MICU spent as CAM+. Although no statistical significance was established relative to the small sample size, the pilot study results indicated the MUSIC group (n = 3) experienced less proportion of time CAM+ (33%) than the control group (n = 3) did (67%). The pilot study design is easily reproducible for larger sample sizes and across multiple units and/or organizations, and it required no additional training or time for staff. The resources needed to provide the prescribed dosing intervals of therapeutic music listening were already available in every patient room. All members of the HCT were actively engaged in the process from inception to completion.

There were several limitations to this pilot study, including the small sample size, time constraints, competing research studies, patient and family self-selection, and single-site unit versus multiple ICUs and patient populations. The small sample size was affected by the time constraints and competing research studies. This pilot study was performed over a 2-week period, which coincided with a large randomized clinical

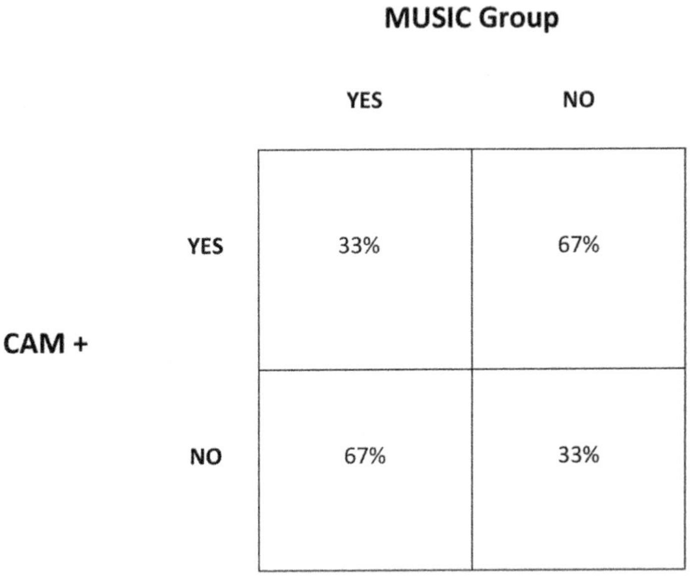

MUSIC Group

	YES	NO
YES	33%	67%
NO	67%	33%

CAM +

Fig. 4. MUSIC group.

trial that was being funded by the National Institutes of Health (NIH). The NIH-funded research study clinicians were enrolling MV patients within the same MICU and the problem of interest was ICU delirium. This meant that all the patients who were enrolled in this pilot study had already declined to participate in the NIH study, which provided blinded pharmaceutical intervention for patients with delirium. The patients and families who declined the NIH study and enrolled in this pilot study could have contributed to confounding factors, resulting in skewed data because perhaps those patients and families did not agree with the use of pharmaceutical products and preferred natural therapies. Another limitation included the use of a single ICU versus multiple ICU patient populations.

Prescribed dosing intervals of therapeutic music do not interfere with activities of daily living and may motivate patients to participate.[36] Anecdotally, colloquialism seemed to affect the patients' music selections and may be worth exploring in future studies. Two of the three MUSIC group patients selected bluegrass, country, and gospel genres, which are popular in the region where this pilot study was performed. Shared decision-making with patients and families and considering their values, beliefs, and needs, clinicians create the best outcomes based on what the patients and families deem most important.[31,32] Enrolling the patients through their families and asking the families to provide the patients' preferred music genre, the families shared in the decision-making process while also keeping the patients' values and beliefs at the forefront of their decision-making.

There is the additional benefit to clinicians of forming therapeutic relationships with the patients and families by providing the patients with an intervention that is specifically tailored to their choice of music. Delivery of holistic care to the patients allows family members to feel a sense of respect, trust, and support while the patients are in the ICU.[37,38] Nursing research has proved to advance unconventional treatment in the setting of removing specific interventions and replacing them wholly with alternative interventions.[39] Consequently, no additional time or resource demands of the nursing staff will contribute to nurse satisfaction, which is invaluable to both health care and patients.[39] The findings of this study support continued effort focused on providing patients and families with focused, personalized, and meaningful care while also allowing clinicians to provide inexpensive and patient-specific interventions aimed at decreasing health care costs associated with morbidity and mortality related to MV and delirium.

DEDICATION

In Honor of Dr Arthur "Art" Wheeler

Those of us who had the great privilege of knowing Art will all agree, he was special. One of a kind human and physician, really. He was the ultimate advocate for people...patients, physicians, and especially nurses. He was a dreamer, a believer, brilliant in so many ways, but mostly he loved life and his exuberance was contagious to everyone around him. I am forever thankful for my time with Art and for his encouragement, guidance, support, and the value he placed on establishing and maintaining a culture of team throughout the medical center and university. Without his clinical and research expertise, leadership, mentorship, and participation as one of my pilot study committee co-chairs, this pilot study could not have come to fruition. His lessons will continue to resonate with so many of us in health care, and I hope we continue to honor him by valuing all he taught us. Be compassionate. Advocate for patients and for each other. And lastly, accomplish great things together and do so with the wonder and excitement that is fitting of exploration and new discoveries.

ACKNOWLEDGMENTS

The authors would like to acknowledge the contributions of Arthur P. "Art" Wheeler, M.D., FCCP (posthumous), who was a Professor of Medicine at Vanderbilt University and Director of Adult Medical Intensive Care Unit for Vanderbilt University Medical Center, and Cathy Cooper EDD, MSN, RN, who is an Associate Professor of School of Nursing at Vanderbilt University.

DISCLOSURE

The authors and contributors have no relationships with commercial companies that have a direct financial interest in subject matter or materials discussed in this article or with companies making competing products.

REFERENCES

1. Pratt RR, Jones RW. Music and medicine: a partnership in history. Berlin: Springer; 1987. https://doi.org/10.1007/978-3-642-71697-3_36.
2. Cui MH, Opoku Agyeman M, Knox D. A crosscultural study of music in history. Int J Cult Hist 2016;2(2):65–9.
3. Mofredj A, Alaya S, Tassaioust K, et al. Music therapy, a review of the potential therapeutic benefits for the critically ill. J Crit Care 2016;35:195–9.
4. Bradt J, Dileo C. Music interventions for mechanically ventilated patients. Cochrane Database Syst Rev 2014;12:1–73.
5. Lee O, Chung Y, Chan M, et al. Music and its effect on the physiological responses and anxiety levels of patients receiving mechanical ventilation: A pilot study. J Clin Nurs 2005;14(5):609–20.
6. Definition and Quotes about Music Therapy. 2019. Available at: musictherapy. org; https://www.musictherapy.org/about/quotes/. Accessed August 14, 2019.
7. Golino AJ, Leone R, Gollenberg A, et al. Impact of an active music therapy intervention on intensive care patients. Am J Crit Care 2019;28(1):48–55.
8. Hunter B, Oliva R, Sahler O, et al. Music therapy as an adjunctive treatment in the management of stress for patients being weaned from mechanical ventilation. J Music Ther 2010;47(3):198–219.
9. Korhan E, Khorshid L, Uyar M. The effect of music therapy on physiological signs of anxiety in patients receiving mechanical ventilatory support. J Clin Nurs 2011; 20(7–8):1026–34.
10. Chlan L, Weinert C, Heiderscheit A, et al. Effects of patient-directed music intervention on anxiety and sedative exposure in critically ill patients receiving mechanical ventilator support: A randomized clinical trial. J Am Med Assoc 2013; 309(22):2335–44.
11. Hayhurst CJ, Pandharipande PP, Hughes CG. Intensive care unit delirium: A review of diagnosis, prevention, and treatment. Anesthesiology 2016;125(6): 1229–41.
12. Dasta J, Kane-Gill S, Pencina M, et al. A cost-minimization analysis of dexmedetomidine compared with midazolam for long-term sedation in the intensive care unit. Crit Care Med 2010;38(2):497–503.
13. Milbrandt E, Deppen S, Harrison P, et al. Costs associated with delirium in mechanically ventilated patients. Crit Care Med 2004;32(4):955–62.
14. Van Den Boogaard M, Schoonhoven L, Hoeven J, et al. Incidence and short-term consequences of delirium in critically ill patients: A prospective observational cohort study. Int J Nurs Stud 2011;49(7):775–83.

15. Boot R. Delirium: A review of the nurses role in the intensive care. Intensive Crit Care Nurs 2011;28(3):185–9.
16. Ely E, Shintani A, Truman B, et al. Delirium as a predictor of mortality in mechanically ventilated patients in the intensive care unit. J Am Med Assoc 2014;291(14): 1753–62.
17. Salluh JIF, Wang H, Schneider EB, et al. Outcome of delirium in critically ill patients: Systematic review and meta-analysis. BMJ 2015;350:h2538.
18. American Association of Critical-Care Nurses. AACN practice alerts: Delirium assessment and management. Crit Care Nurse 2012;32(1):79–82.
19. Hsieh JS, Ely WE, Gong MN. Can intensive care unit delirium be prevented and reduced? Lessons learned and future directions. Ann Am Thorac Soc 2013;10(6): 648–56.
20. Neufeld KJ. American delirium society. 2016. Available at: https:// americandeliriumsociety.org/blog/pharmacologic-approaches-managing- delirium. Accessed August 16, 2019.
21. Cavalazzi R, Saad M, Marik P. Delirium in the ICU: an overview. Ann Intensive Care 2012;2(49):1–11.
22. Confusion assessment method for the ICU (CAM-ICU). Vanderbilt University Medical Center. 2019. Available at: https://www.icudelirium.org/medical- professionals/downloads/resources-by-category. Accessed March 4, 2019.
23. Sessler C, Gosnell M, Grap M, et al. The Richmond agitation-sedation scale: Validity and reliability in adult intensive care unit patients. Am J Respir Crit Care Med 2002;166(10):1338–44.
24. Ely EW, Truman B, Shintani A, et al. Monitoring sedation status over time in ICU patients: Reliability and validity of the Richmond agitation-sedation scale (RASS). JAMA 2003;289(22):2983–91.
25. Khan BA, Perkins AJ, Gao S, et al. The CAM-ICU-7 delirium severity scale: A novel delirium severity instrument for use in the intensive care unit. Crit Care Med 2017;45(5):851–7.
26. Gélinas C, Bérubé M, Chevrier A, et al. Delirium assessment tools for use in critically ill adults: A psychometric analysis and systematic review. Crit Care Nurse 2018;38(1):38–50.
27. Miranda F, Arevalo-Rodriguez I, Díaz G, et al. Confusion Assessment Method for the intensive care unit (CAM-ICU) for the diagnosis of delirium in adults in critical care settings. Cochrane Database Syst Rev 2018;(9):CD013126.
28. McCormack B, McCance T. Person-centred nursing: theory and practice. Oxford (United Kingdom): Wiley-Blackwell; 2010.
29. McCormack B, McCance T. Development of a framework for person-centred nursing. J Adv Nurs 2006;56(5):472–9.
30. Barry M, Edgman-Levitan S. Shared decision making: The pinnacle of patient- centered care. N Engl J Med 2012;366:780–1.
31. Kelley K. The patient self-determination act: A matter of life and death. Physician Assist 1995;53(6):59–60.
32. Tracy M, Chlan L, Staugaitis A. Perceptions of patients and families who received a music intervention during mechanical ventilation. Music Med 2015;7(3):54–8.
33. Brummel NE, Boehm LM, Girard TD, et al. Subsyndromal delirium and institutionalization among patients with critical illness. Am J Crit Care 2017;26(6):447–55.
34. Ely EW. CAM-ICU Training Manual. Monitoring Delirium in the ICU. 2016. Available at: icudelirium.org; https://www.icudelirium.org/medical-professionals/ delirium/monitoring-delirium-in-the-icu. Accessed January 25, 2020.

35. Spronk P, Riekirk B, Hofhuis J, et al. Occurrence of delirium is severely underestimated in the ICU during daily care. Intensive Care Med 2009;35(7):1276–80.
36. Boldt S. The effects of music therapy on motivation, psychological well-being, physical comfort, and exercise endurance of bone marrow transplant patients. J Music Ther 1996;33(3):164–88.
37. McCaffrey R, Locsin R. Music listening as a nursing intervention: A symphony of practice. Holist Nurs Pract 2002;16(3):70–7.
38. Mitchell M, Chaboyer W, Burmeister E, et al. Positive effects of a nursing intervention on family-centered care in adult critical care. Am J Crit Care 2009;18(6):543–52.
39. Fagin C. The economic value of nursing research. Am J Nurs 1982;82(12):1844–9.

Efficacy of Acupuncture/ Acupressure in the Prevention and Treatment of Nausea and Vomiting Across Multiple Patient Populations
Implications for Practice

Angela Morehead, DNP, FNP-BC, RN*,
Garrett Salmon, DNP, RN, CRNA, APN

KEYWORDS

- Nausea • Vomiting • Acupuncture • Acupressure • Postoperative • Pregnancy

KEY POINTS

- Nausea and vomiting are complex symptoms that can be related to many disease processes.
- Providers should be encouraged to provide the patient with all information regarding efficacy and side effects of acupuncture and acupressure related to nausea and vomiting.
- Providers should discuss the potential out of pocket cost that could be incurred due to lack of insurance coverage of alternative treatments.

DIAGNOSIS/ASSESSMENT

Nausea and vomiting is extremely complex, and involves the physiologic state, gastrointestinal system, central nervous system, and autonomic nervous system.[1] Neurons in the brainstem comprise the medullary reticular formation, and these neurons are activated by irritation of the vagal and other nerves in the in the pharynx, heart, peritoneum, mesentery, bile ducts, stomach, and bowel.[1] The vomiting center is activated by the nucleus tractus solitarius, or "relay station" in the brain, when noxious stimuli or toxins are present.[1] The experience of nausea and vomiting also includes an autonomic nervous system response that leads to sweating, pallor, salivation, increased blood pressure, tachycardia, and cutaneous vasoconstriction.[1]

School of Nursing, Middle Tennessee State University, Box 81, Murfreesboro, TN 37132, USA
* Corresponding author.
E-mail address: Angela.Morehead@mtsu.edu

Nurs Clin N Am 55 (2020) 571–580
https://doi.org/10.1016/j.cnur.2020.07.001
0029-6465/20/© 2020 Elsevier Inc. All rights reserved.

The Rome criteria was developed in 1988 in an effort to classify gastrointestinal disorders. The criteria allow clinicians to diagnose disorders by grouping self-reported symptoms into syndromes, and can help to guide clinicians in the treatment of these disorders based on the pathophysiology, which includes disorders of motility, hypersensitivity, or brain-gut dysfunction.[2] In 2015, the fourth iteration of the Rome criteria was approved.[2] The subcategory of nausea and vomiting is included under gastroduodenal disorders, and includes chronic nausea vomiting syndrome, cyclic vomiting syndrome, and cannabinoid hyperemesis syndrome.[2]

CHRONIC AND ACUTE NAUSEA AND VOMITING

Chronic nausea can be related to multiple etiologies, including gastroesophageal reflux, gastroparesis, and vertigo. Chronic nausea and vomiting is categorized as symptoms that are present for more than 1 month, and can be challenging to diagnose because of the difficulty in narrowing down a specific cause.[3] This type of nausea and vomiting is typically evaluated in an outpatient setting, and can also be related to nystagmus or bulimia, among other disorders of the gut, peritoneal cavity, or central nervous system.[3,4]

Acute nausea can be caused by migraine headache, chemotherapy, early pregnancy, and chronic cannabinoid use.[4] Acute vomiting, which is categorized as vomiting lasting for hours to several days, can be related to viral gastroenteritis, bowel obstruction, drug use, including cannabis and opioids, migraine headache, or early pregnancy.[4] Acute vomiting of coffee ground material can indicate gastrointestinal bleeding, and vomiting accompanied by abdominal pain can indicate cholecystitis.[5]

PHARMACOLOGIC TREATMENT OF NAUSEA AND VOMITING

Treatment of nausea and vomiting is dependent on many factors. The etiology of the nausea and vomiting should be investigated, and any sequelae should be corrected (electrolyte imbalance and dehydration).[4] Medications are used based on severity of symptoms and the cause of the nausea and vomiting, with the most commonly prescribed pharmacologic interventions for nausea and vomiting including antiemetics, prokinetics, antihistamines, and phenothiazines.[1,4] Antiemetics, including ondansetron and granisetron, prevent nausea and vomiting by central nervous system action. Prokinetics, including erythromycin, decrease nausea by acting on the stomach to increase the rate of gastric emptying.[1] If the patient has nausea and vomiting from a vestibular issue, including "motion sickness," antihistamines, such as promethazine and meclizine, are used due to their central anticholinergic effects.[1]

The recommended pharmacologic treatment for common causes of nausea and vomiting is outlined in **Table 1**.[4]

Table 1
Recommended pharmacologic treatment for common causes of nausea and vomiting

Diagnosis	Recommended Treatment
Migraine headache	Metoclopramide, prochlorperazine, oral antiemetic, serotonin antagonists
Vestibular nausea (from inner ear, vertigo)	Antihistamine, anticholinergics
Gastroenteritis	Dopamine antagonists, serotonin antagonists

Data from Longstreth, G. Approach to the adult with nausea and vomiting. UptoDate. Retrieved March 1, 2020.

The use of pharmacologic interventions for nausea and vomiting is not without risk. The antiemetic medications that work primarily as 5-HT$_3$ antagonists (ondansetron and granisetron) have been associated with torsades de pointe.[1] Metoclopramide, a benzamide that works as a 5-HT$_3$ and D$_2$ receptor antagonist, has been noted to cause extrapyramidal effects, including tardive dyskinesia.[1]

Although nausea and vomiting can be a protective mechanism against ingested toxins, it can lead to many problems, including electrolyte imbalance, dehydration, and weight loss.[6] The cost of nausea and vomiting due to gastrointestinal infection to the health care system exceeds $3.4 billion every year, and this does not include the cost associated with other causes of nausea and vomiting.[6] Costs of medical testing, as well as lost work time, adds to this expense.[6] This is especially relevant for pregnant women and their employers; an average of 62 hours of missed work can be due to nausea and vomiting from pregnancy.[6] Patients who suffer from migraines with associated nausea and vomiting have been found to use the emergency room more often than those who do not have nausea and vomiting, and have 26% higher cost associated with their migraines.[7]

WHAT IS ACUPUNCTURE?

Acupuncture is the use of thin needles to stimulate specific places on the body.[1,8] This traditional Chinese technique is thought to balance the flow of energy.[9] In Eastern medicine, disease is considered to be an imbalance, and how organs and tissues work together is considered to be the way to balance health.[10] One theory explaining the mechanism by which acupuncture works is the gate theory of pain.[10] The theory is that acupuncture initiates inhibitory signals that effectively negate stimulatory signals.[10] Another theory for the mechanism of action is that acupuncture stimulates the release of endorphins and endogenous opioids, and alters the opioid receptors in the brain.[10] Traditional Chinese medicine posits the theory that PC6 acupoint stimulation regulates the function of the stomach qi and subsequently prevents nausea and vomiting.[11] More recent literature has hypothesized that the antiemetic effect of acupuncture stems from the resulted increase in hypophyseal secretion of beta-endorphins and adrenocorticotropic hormone (ACTH), with subsequent inhibition of the chemoreceptor trigger zone (CTZ) and vomiting center.[10]

The body is divided into 14 meridians, and there are more than 2000 acupuncture points along these meridians.[10] Each of these points has a specific quality to restore balance.[10]

The clinician places the needles in 5 to 15 points on the body based on the assessment, and the needles are inserted millimeters to 2 to 3 cm deep.[10] The Food and Drug Administration regulates acupuncturists, or those practitioners providing acupuncture, and most states require that an acupuncturist take and pass a certifying examination.[9]

Many patients have reported relief from multiple conditions, including headache, low back pain, and arthritis pain.[8] Acupuncture has also been studied extensively for treatment of depression and for smoking cessation, but there is conflicting evidence regarding the efficacy for these issues.[8] It has also been reviewed for treatment of menopause symptoms and overactive bladder, and although the results demonstrated benefits with these symptoms, the data were limited.[10]

When compared with pharmacologic interventions, acupuncture has relatively few side effects or complications. Adverse events have been noted to occur most often when an acupuncturist is not trained properly, or when the needles that are used have not been properly sterilized,[8] with insertion site infection being the most commonly reported adverse event.[10] More serious, but unlikely, adverse events also include pneumothorax, nervous system injury, and peripheral nerve injury.[10] Rare reports of numbness or tingling at the insertion site, bleeding, and bruising have been noted, and patients should be counseled that although for some conditions there is a lack of evidence regarding efficacy, the risk of acupuncture is minimal.[10]

Another advantage of acupuncture compared with pharmacologic treatment is that there are few contraindications to the use of acupuncture. Those patients with a bleeding disorder and those with a pacemaker should be carefully evaluated before acupuncture, and providers are encouraged to be aware that some acupuncture points could induce preterm labor in the pregnant patient.[9]

WHAT IS ACUPRESSURE?

Acupressure is the use of manual pressure on the same points that are used in acupuncture treatment.[12] The use of acupressure is noninvasive and is essentially free of side effects.[12]

The exact mechanism of action of acupressure is unknown, but there are several theories. The use of low-frequency transcutaneous stimulation has been found to alter transmission of neurotransmitters.[13] Another theory is that acupressure alters gastric acid secretions.[13] The most common acupressure points are the pericardium 6 (PC6) area, located two-thumb widths above the distal crease of the internal wrist, and the KID21 point that is located approximately 2.5 inches below the sternocostal angle.[13]

Acupressure has been demonstrated to be efficacious for nausea and vomiting, and is considered to be safe.[13] It is noninvasive, and has no known side effects[12] (**Box 1**).

BACKGROUND

There are approximately 30 million anesthetics administered each year in the United States, or approximately 10% of the population.[14] With this large number of anesthetics also comes the risk for a patient to experience what is known as postoperative nausea and vomiting (PONV). Postoperative nausea and vomiting is a condition that can be present after the administration of anesthesia and surgery. PONV has an overall incidence rate of 40% to 90%.[15] PONV is defined as any nausea, retching, or vomiting occurring during the first 24 to 48 hours after surgery.[5] PONV is not only known as one of the highest reasons for patient dissatisfaction after anesthesia, it has other negative side effects as well. PONV accounts for up to 80% of postoperative complications, and antiemetic drug therapy is not only costly but can cause side effects such as sedation and headache.[11] PONV is not only problematic for patients in that it can

---

Box 1
Acupuncture in the prevention of postoperative induced nausea and vomiting (PONV) and chemotherapy

1. Background on postoperative nausea and vomiting (PONV)
2. PC6 acupuncture's clinical efficacy in prevention of PONV
3. Application to common general surgery procedures (eg, laparoscopic cholecystectomy)
4. Female-specific surgical cases (eg, mastectomy, gynecologic procedures)
5. Pediatric-specific surgical case application (eg, tonsillectomy)
6. Chemotherapy-induced nausea and vomiting treatment

negatively affect their recovery from surgery, but it increases costs to the health care system due to prolonged hospital stays and unanticipated readmissions.[11]

PERICARDIUM 6 ACUPUNCTURE'S CLINICAL EFFICACY IN PREVENTION OF POSTOPERATIVE NAUSEA AND VOMITING

To help combat the incidence of PONV, recent advances in the usage of acupuncture/acupressure have been investigated as an alternative to current pharmacologic treatments. In relation to acupuncture, a vast majority of research has focused on examining the efficacy of stimulation of the wrist at the "Pericardium (PC6) acupuncture point" to reduce nausea and vomiting, although the process by which this intervention specifically prevents PONV has not been established in Western medicine. Research has noted that in a review of 6 pooled studies (580 participants) the usage of PC6 acupuncture resulted in a 30.8% incidence of PONV versus 43.4% for the control group, which had no previous intervention.[15] Another analysis was conducted using a large review of the Cochrane database, which encompassed 59 trials that were conducted between 1986 and 2015, involving 7677 patients who received elective surgery, 7 of which were conducted with 727 pediatric patients. This analysis found that when compared with SHAM treatment, which is placebo, that PC6 acupoint stimulation produced a clinically significant beneficial effect in reducing the incidence of nausea, vomiting, and the need for recue antiemetics.[11]

Time of application of acupuncture and its relation to the clinical efficacy is also important to note when educating patients experiencing nausea and vomiting. Because acupuncture is not a drug, its effects are not immediate, and reapplication to increase efficacy and duration of this intervention is a critical component of success. Research has noted that patients who received PC6 acupuncture 30 minutes before and up to 72 hours after surgery significantly increased the complete responses to treatment (68%) compared with before surgery only (43%).[15] It is also important to note the amount of time it takes for the procedure of acupuncture to take place. In the vast majority of research that was evaluated, it is commonly agreed on that optimal time over which the PC6 acupuncture is to take place is for 1 minute of initial bead compression, with 2 additional 30-second presses over the next 5 minutes, which achieved an 87% complete response versus other timing techniques.[15]

With the background of PONV and the usage of acupuncture as an alternative to current pharmacologic treatment being introduced, a more in-depth look at specific surgical patient populations in relation to clinical efficacy of this intervention is needed.

APPLICATION TO COMMON GENERAL SURGERY PROCEDURES

With regard to application of acupuncture in surgical patients, it is important to examine the utility of this technique, when applied to the more commonly occurring procedures in this patient population. The most often performed general surgery procedure in the United States is the laparoscopic cholecystectomy, with approximately 130 being performed per 100,000 people each year.[16] As previously discussed, the surgical patient population is at a high risk for development PONV due to the combined effects of surgical and anesthetic requirements necessary for surgical conditions. A double-blind, randomized controlled trial of 56 patients who were assigned to separate acupuncture and placebo groups found that postoperatively 48.2% in the placebo group experienced PONV, whereas none was experienced in the acupuncture group.[17] The clinical implications of this research showed that PC6 stimulation is a viable technique to prevent PONV, with minimal risk or side effects in patients within this common surgical population.

FEMALE AND PEDIATRIC-SPECIFIC SURGICAL CASE APPLICATION

Another subset of surgical patients that could potentially benefit from the application of acupuncture are those who are pediatric or female. These patients have very specific risk factors for PONV that do not fall within normal occurrence. Female patients who undergo surgical procedures involving the breasts or gynecologic procedures are at a significantly increased risk of experiencing PONV, due to increased activation of the CTZ.[18]

Given the potential for complications that can occur as a result of PONV that were previously discussed, it is not surprising that this patient population is of particular importance when discussing prevention and treatment options. A study conducted by Quinlan-Woodward et. al.[18] used a randomized, double-blind analysis of female patients who underwent surgical mastectomy (ie, unilteral simple mastectomy, bilateral simple mastectomy, and bilateral extended mastectomy), in which the findings showed that patients who were placed in the acupuncture group showed statistically significantly less nausea postoperatively (P = .011) than the control group, who received standard pharmacologic treatment. This research showed acupuncture as a safe and effective alternative to traditional treatment regimens in this highly at-risk subpopulation of patients.

With regard to pediatric patients, the conversation changes somewhat in the utilization of acupuncture to prevent PONV. In this patient population, the postoperative complications of PONV with more common procedures (such as tonsillectomy) present a different and more immediate risk to the patient. Nineteen percent of children who underwent adenotonsillectomy experienced a postoperative complication, with 9.4% experiencing respiratory compromise, the most frequent complication, and 2.6% having secondary hemorrhage, according to a meta-analysis.[19] It also of note that the presence of PONV in these patients was said to play a direct role in the occurrence rate of these complications due to increased pressure on tissues that had surgically cauterized, causing them to swell and hemorrhage.[19] Because airway hemorrhage and swelling can directly lead to airway compromise, it is imperative to mitigate the risk of this occurrence. A meta-analysis conducted by Shin and colleagues,[20] who selected 8 articles for review (4 randomized controlled trials, 3 prospective cohorts, and 1 pilot study) revealed that the number of patients with PONV was significantly reduced with acupuncture compared with the control group, with a risk ratio of 0.77 (95% confidence interval: 0.63–0.94, $P<.05$). In this instance, the risk of postoperative complications such as respiratory compromise and hemorrhage are largely negated with the usage of acupuncture in comparison with traditional pharmacologic treatment.

CHEMOTHERAPY AND ACUPUNCTURE

Nausea and vomiting are frequent side effects associated with chemotherapy treatments. This incidence is largely contributed to the emetic potential of the drugs used in chemotherapy. Approximately 30% of chemotherapeutic agents induce significant nausea and vomiting.[21] The symptoms related to nausea and vomiting can occur at 3 different times: (1) during the anticipation that occurs before administration of chemotherapy; (2) immediately or acutely, up to 24 hours after infusion; and (3) late, occurring 24 hours after the administration of chemotherapy and lasting for 4 to 5 days.[21] With regard to chemotherapy, the overall goal of antiemetic therapy is to reduce or prevent nausea and vomiting, which will allow patients to maintain adequate hydration and take in food, which helps to preserve quality of life while circumventing possible electrolyte disorders, malnutrition, and dehydration. Despite the currently available antiemetic therapies, gastrointestinal disorders affect between 45% and 75% of patients receiving antineoplastic treatments.[21]

A recent study was conducted using a randomized controlled format in which 17 patients were given acupuncture for 1 minute on days 1, 2, 3, and 5 of each chemotherapy cycle, and overall the results represented a total of 52 chemotherapy cycles. The results of the study showed that the group that received acupuncture had an occurrence rate of nausea and vomiting that was between 4% and 19% during days 1 through 5 after chemotherapy, versus the control group, which showed an occurrence rate of nausea and vomiting of 28% to 51% during the corresponding time period. The results of this study showed that acupuncture was effective at relieving vomiting and nausea during the 5-day period after chemotherapy.[21]

Another study, by Xie and colleagues,[22] showed that the usage of acupuncture was a safe and effective therapy to relieve patients' gastrointestinal discomfort after chemotherapy for hepatic cancer, when measured out to a time of 5 days after treatment versus the control group. It is also worth noting as with other previously discussed studies that the safety and tolerability of acupuncture is very well tolerated by patients in the subpopulation of chemotherapy-induced nausea and vomiting without any mention of negative side effects (**Box 2**).

NAUSEA AND VOMITING IN PREGNANCY

Nausea and vomiting occurs in approximately 50% to 80% of all pregnant women, and if it is persistent can lead to malnutrition.[23] The cause of nausea and vomiting in pregnancy is unknown, but it has been attributed to hormone changes that occur in the first trimester.[13] The most severe form of persistent nausea and vomiting, or hyperemesis gravidarum, is diagnosed when the pregnant patient has a 5% or greater loss of body weight, dehydration, ketosis, and electrolyte imbalance.[4,23] Low income, low education level, history of premenstrual syndrome, and unwanted pregnancy are all risk factors for nausea and vomiting in pregnancy.[13] The economic consequences for pregnancy-related nausea and vomiting, including hospitalization, medications, and other indirect costs exceeded $1 billion in 2012.[24]

Current nonpharmacologic recommendations for treatment of nausea and vomiting in pregnancy include small, frequent meals, eating dry carbohydrates on waking, decreasing fatty or other foods that seem to contribute to nausea and vomiting, and smoking cessation.[25]

Pharmacotherapy for nausea and vomiting in pregnancy includes vitamins, antihistamines, anticholinergics, dopamine antagonists, phenothiazines, butyrophenones, serotonin antagonists, and corticosteroids.[25] Few of these options are approved by the Food and Drug Administration, and many of these medications are used "off-label" for nausea and vomiting.[25]

Box 2
Acupuncture for prevention of nausea and vomiting in pregnancy

1. Background on nausea and vomiting in pregnancy

2. Pharmacologic therapy

3. Complementary therapies

4. Acupressure

5. Acupuncture

With more than 87% of women admitting to use of a complementary therapy for nausea and vomiting during pregnancy,[13] it is essential explore the efficacy and safety of alternatives to pharmacotherapy. The use of complementary therapy for relief of nausea and vomiting in pregnancy is found more frequently in women who have a higher level of education and in those women who have had a vaginal delivery.[13] Common alternative treatments for pregnancy-related nausea and vomiting include ginger, chamomile, peppermint, raspberry tea,[25] cardamom, and lemon.[13]

The use of acupressure at 2 thumb widths above the distal crease of the internal wrist, or PC6 area (Nei Guan point), has been demonstrated to reduce pregnancy related nausea and vomiting.[13] Studies done comparing nausea and vomiting symptoms with the use of manual pressure on the PC6 area (intervention group) compared with a "dummy" spot demonstrated report of decreased symptoms in the intervention group.[26]

The antiemetic effect from acupressure also can be achieved by a pressure wristband on the same pressure point.[25] It should be noted that patients who choose to wear a pressure band demonstrated decreased nausea and vomiting when the band was worn for 24 hours as opposed to 8 hours.[12] Adlan and colleagues[12] also demonstrated improvement in secondary outcomes, including length of hospital stay, ketonuria, and patient satisfaction, with the use of acupressure for nausea and vomiting in pregnancy.

The use of acupuncture for nausea and vomiting in pregnancy also includes the PC6 pressure point. Acupuncture has been demonstrated in some studies to improve nausea and vomiting symptoms in pregnancy, but the evidence is conflicting.[10] A 2018 review of interventions, including acupuncture compared with placebo and metoclopramide, yielded positive results, however, when acupuncture was compared in another study with metoclopramide, there was no reported difference in nausea and vomiting.[10] The pregnant women in the first study who used acupuncture required less antiemetic treatment.[10] Another review demonstrated that acupuncture was effective for nausea and vomiting in pregnancy for patients who were not under the effects of anesthesia.[10]

It is important to note that women who choose acupressure and acupuncture for treatment of nausea and vomiting in pregnancy typically pay out of pocket due to lack of insurance coverage for alternative treatments.[10] Although some commercial or private pay insurances offer coverage for these services, most Medicare plans do not. Providers who recommend alternative treatments should discuss all risks and possible benefits with the patient, and present all evidence related to the efficacy of these treatments.

IMPLICATIONS FOR RESEARCH

With more patients seeking alternative treatments with a lower side-effect profile for nausea and vomiting, continued research related to acupuncture and acupressure are necessary. Larger trials in patients receiving chemotherapy are especially relevant due to high rate of symptoms in these patients and the limited numbers of patients in the studies that have been done. Limitations in the use of pharmacotherapy for pregnancy-related nausea and vomiting warrant the need for additional research of the use of acupressure and acupuncture because these therapies have minimal to no side effects for the pregnant patient.

IMPLICATIONS FOR PRACTICE

Providers should be encouraged to provide the patient with all information regarding efficacy and side effects of acupuncture and acupressure related to nausea and vomiting. In addition, they should discuss the potential out-of-pocket cost that could be incurred due to lack of insurance coverage of alternative treatments.

DISCLOSURE

The authors have nothing to disclose.

REFERENCES

1. Cangemi D, Kuo B. Practical perspectives in the treatment of nausea and vomiting. J Clin Gastroenterol 2019;53(3):170–6.
2. Schmulson MJ, Drossman DA. What is new in Rome IV. J Neurogastroenterol Motil 2017;23(2):151–63.
3. Quigley E, Hasler W, Parkman H. AGA technical review on nausea and vomiting. Gastroenterology 2001;120(1):263–86.
4. Longstreth GF. Approach to the adult with nausea and vomiting. UptoDate; 2020.
5. Pierre S, Whelan R. Nausea and vomiting after surgery. Br J Anaesth 2013;13(1): 28–32.
6. Scorza K, Williams A, Phillips D, et al. Evaluation of nausea and vomiting. Am Fam Physician 2007;76(1):76–84.
7. Gajria K, Lee LK, Flores NM, et al. Humanistic and economic burden of nausea and vomiting among migraine sufferers. J Pain Res 2017;10:689–98.
8. Acupuncture: in depth. 2016. Available at: https://nccih.nih.gov/health/ acupuncture/introduction#hed3. Accessed March 7, 2020.
9. Acupuncture. 2017. Available at: https://www.mayoclinic.org/tests-procedures/ acupuncture/about/pac-20392763. Accessed March 7, 2020.
10. Bishop K, Ford A, Kuller J, et al. Acupuncture in obstetrics and gynecology. Obstet Gynecol Surv 2019;74(4):241–51.
11. Stott A. Examining the efficacy of stimulating the PC6 wrist acupuncture point for preventing postoperative nausea and vomiting: a Cochrane review summary. Int J Nurs Stud 2016;64:139–41.
12. Adlan A, Chooi K, Adenan N. Acupressure as adjuvant treatment for the inpatient management of nausea and vomiting in early pregnancy: a double blind randomized controlled trial. J Obstet Gynaecol Res 2017;43(4):662–8.
13. Ozgoli G, Naz M. Effects of complementary medicine on nausea and vomiting in pregnancy: a systematic review. Int J Prev Med 2018;9:75.
14. Malignant Hyperthermia Association of the United States (MHAUS). How many actually experience an MH episode? How many people are at risk for MH?. Available at: https://www.mhaus.org/blog/how-many-actually-experience-an-mh-episode-how-many-people-are-at-risk-for-mh1/. Accessed February 21, 2020.
15. Cheong KB, Zhang J-p, Huang Y, et al. The effectiveness of acupuncture in the prevention and treatment of postoperative nausea and vomiting-a systematic review and meta-analysis. PLoS One 2013;8(12):1–17.
16. Most frequent operating room procedures performed in U.S. hospitals, 2003-2012. Healthcare Cost and Utilization Project (HCUP). 2014. Available at: https://www.hcup-us.ahrq.gov/reports/statbriefs/sb186-Operating-Room-Procedures-United-States-2012.jsp. Accessed March 9, 2020.
17. Carr KL, Johnson FE, Kenaan CA, et al. Effects of P6 stimulation of postoperative nausea and vomiting in laparoscopic cholecystectomy patients. J Perianesth Nurs 2015;30(3):328.

18. Quinlan-Woodward J, Gode A, Dusek JA, et al. Assessing the impact of acupuncture on pain, nausea, anxiety and coping in women undergoing a mastectomy. Oncol Nurs Forum 2016;43(6):725–32.
19. One fifth of kids have complication after tonsillectomy. Medscape. 2015. Available at: https://www.medscape.com/viewarticle/851386. Accessed March 10, 2020.
20. Shin H, Kim J, Lee S, et al. The effect of acupuncture on postoperative nausea and vomiting after pediatric tonsillectomy: A meta-analysis and systematic review. Laryngoscope 2016;126(8):1761–7.
21. Varejao C, Santo F. Laser acupuncture for relieving nausea and vomiting in pediatric patients undergoing chemotherapy: A single-blind randomized clinical trial. J Pediatr Oncol Nurs 2019;36(1):44–54.
22. Xie J, Chen L, Ning Z, et al. Effect of transcutaneous electrical acupoint stimulation combined with palonosetron on chemotherapy-induced nausea and vomiting: a single-blind randomized, controlled trial. Chin J Cancer 2017;36:6.
23. Van del Heuvel E, Goosens M, Vanderhaegen H, et al. Effect of acustimulation on nausea and vomiting and on hyperemesis in pregnancy; a systematic review of Western and Chinese literature. BMC Complement Altern Med 2016;16:13.
24. Khorasani F, Aryan H, Sobhi A, et al. A systematic review of the efficacy of alternative medicine in the treatment of nausea and vomiting in pregnancy. J Obstet Gynecol 2019;40(1):10–9.
25. Argenbright C. Complementary approaches to pregnancy induced nausea and vomiting. Int J Childbirth Educ 2017;32(1):6–8.
26. Roscoe J, Matteson S. Acupressure and acustimulation bands for control of nausea: a brief review. Am J Obstet Gynecol 2002;186(5):S244–7.

Health Benefits of Tai Chi Exercise: A Guide for Nurses

Sally M. Miller, PhD, RN[a],*, Cindy Hui-Lio, EdD[b,c],
Ruth E. Taylor-Piliae, PhD, RN[d]

KEYWORDS

• Tai chi • Cognition • Depression • Sleep • Heart failure • Stroke • Fall prevention

KEY POINTS

- Tai chi is an ancient Chinese internal martial art that has increased in popularity across the United States over the past 2 decades.
- There is increasing scientific evidence showing the positive impact of tai chi exercise on multifaceted areas of health and well-being.
- Tai chi exercise is associated with several physical and psychological benefits, including improved cognition, less depression and anxiety, better sleep and cardiovascular health, and fewer accidental falls.
- Nurses are in unique positions to recommend tai chi exercise, assist patients to find qualified tai chi instructors, and/or enroll in appropriate tai chi classes.

INTRODUCTION

The World Health Organization (WHO) defines health as more than the absence of disease, and measures physical, mental, and social well-being as indicators of quality of life (QOL).[1] Aligned with this global emphasis on health and well-being is the United States government's Healthy People 2020 initiative, which envisions and measures improvement in the health of Americans, including health-related QOL (HRQoL) and well-being.[2] HRQoL is a multidimensional concept that includes physical, mental, emotional, and social functioning, and well-being is the ability of a person to live a full and satisfying life.[2] HRQoL and well-being can be affected through optimizing physical, mental, and social functioning. Personal lifestyle choices and activities such as exercise have significant impact on a person's health and well-being. One

[a] Vanderbilt University School of Nursing, 461 21st Avenue South, Nashville, TN 37240, USA;
[b] Osher Center for Integrative Medicine at Vanderbilt, Vanderbilt University Medical Center, 3401 West End Avenue, Suite 380, Nashville, TN 37203, USA; [c] Blair School of Music, Vanderbilt University, Nashville, TN, USA; [d] University of Arizona College of Nursing, Room 329, PO Box 210203, Tucson, AZ 85721-0203, USA
* Corresponding author.
E-mail address: sally.m.miller@vanderbilt.edu

Nurs Clin N Am 55 (2020) 581–600
https://doi.org/10.1016/j.cnur.2020.07.002
0029-6465/20/© 2020 Elsevier Inc. All rights reserved.

nursing.theclinics.com

form of exercise with broad positive impacts on physical, mental, and emotional health and social well-being is tai chi exercise.

Tai chi is an ancient Chinese internal martial art that has increased in popularity across the United States over the past decade.[3] There is increasing scientific evidence showing the positive impact of tai chi exercise on multifaceted areas of health and well-being as a safe form of exercise, even among older adults or those with a chronic illness.[4] Tai chi exercise is endorsed by the Centers for Disease Control and Prevention for fall prevention[5] and the National Center for Complementary and Integrative Health/National Institute of Aging[5] both to maintain and improve health and as a complement to therapies for chronic conditions.[6]

Tai chi exercise is characterized by slow, intentional movements, mindfulness, meditative breathing, imagery, and a focus on balance. Tai chi exercise can be done standing, while seated in a chair, or as a combination of the two. Tai chi exercise classes are widely available in many community-based facilities such as senior centers, libraries, or faith-based organizations. Under the guidance of a qualified instructor, this form of exercise is appropriate for people who have been sedentary or those with chronic health conditions. Tai chi exercise can be considered a so-called gateway exercise because of its low impact on joints, its gentle, balanced movements, and its fitness benefits, which then contribute to increased exercise self-efficacy and aerobic endurance. Because of its meditative features, focus on breathing, and aerobic components, tai chi exercise research has documented physical and psychological benefits including positive effects on cognition, depression, anxiety, sleep, cardiovascular health, and fall prevention. In addition, and importantly, tai chi exercise can positively affect QOL because of the individual's engagement in social and leisure activity.

There is existing evidence that shows the benefits of tai chi for improvement and maintenance of physical, mental, and social functioning and as a holistic and complementary adjunct to therapies for chronic health conditions. Mind-body interventions such as tai chi are a growing science, and although there is an acknowledged need for additional rigorous and longitudinal studies, the positive impact of this gentle form of exercise is becoming more evident. In addition to presenting the current body of evidence, this article provides nurses with recommendations to assist patients to find qualified tai chi instructors and/or enroll in appropriate tai chi classes (Appendix 1). These recommendations will assist nurses to articulate the benefits of tai chi and promote this accessible form of exercise with the aim of meeting the multidimensional goals of the WHO and Healthy People 2020 and beyond.

Brain Health and Cognitive Decline

Problem/cause

As the population of the United States ages, cognitive decline is recognized as a growing public health concern. Signs and symptoms of cognitive decline include memory loss, difficulty learning, problems with decision making, and confusion.[7] The Centers for Disease Control and Prevention (CDC) Healthy Brain Initiative focuses on maintaining cognitive health, including reducing the incidence of cognitive decline and promoting scientific discovery related to preserving cognitive function. Promotion of brain-healthy interventions such as physical activity and exercise is part of that mandate.

Current treatment

Physical activity and exercise are known to have beneficial effects on brain health through multiple pathways, including creation of new vasculature, stimulation of hormones to support neural growth, and promotion of brain plasticity.[8] The CDC recommends a minimum of 150 to 300 minutes of moderate-intensity exercise each week for adults. Tai chi is considered a light-to-moderate aerobic exercise with benefits similar to brisk walking[9] and can therefore be included in exercise regimes to meet these requirements. In addition, current guidelines support the benefit of short sessions of moderate-intensity exercise, making tai chi an accessible gateway exercise to increase activity tolerance and reach recommended goals.[10]

Tai chi intervention studies
A recent systematic review and meta-analysis[11] examined 28 studies, including randomized and nonrandomized trials, primarily in adults 60 years of age and older and in people with and without cognitive impairment. The frequency and duration of tai chi interventions ranged from 1 to several times per week, lasting 20 to 120 minutes per session. Intervention groups were compared with Western-type exercise control groups (eg, stretching, resistance training), health education, and nonintervention controls. A positive association between tai chi exercise and executive function was observed in the randomized trials, with evidence to suggest positive effects in other cognitive domains, including language, learning, and/or memory.

Measures
Measures of cognition included global cognition (eg, Mini-Mental State Examination [MMSE]),[12] executive function such as information processing speed and working memory (eg, digit span tests, Stroop color and word tests, trail-making tests), measures of language and verbal fluency (eg, animal naming test, Boston Naming Test), assessment of learning and memory (eg, California Verbal Learning Test, Hong Kong List Learning Test), and spatial and quantitative assessments (eg, clock-drawing test, word problems).[13]

Proposed therapeutic effects
The multimodal and interactive physical, cognitive, and psychological mechanisms inherent in tai chi exercise may contribute to promotion of brain health. There is strong evidence supporting the impact of aerobic exercise on structural brain components, including increased plasticity, vascular generation, and neuronal growth.[8] In addition, tai chi practice includes meditation, memorization of sequences and postures, attentional components, and improved physical fitness. All of these components are associated with improved cognitive function[11] (**Table 1**).

Mental Health: Depression and Anxiety

Problem/cause
Psychological well-being is described as having positive emotions and functioning well in physical, mental, and social domains.[14] Well-being in these domains is negatively affected by conditions such as depression and anxiety. Depression is characterized by prolonged extreme sadness and effects approximately 1 out of every 6 adults in the United States at some time of their lives.[15] Depression disrupts personal relationships, physical health, work productivity, and leisure activity. Anxiety disorders often occur in conjunction with depression and can be psychologically disabling because of persistent feelings of fear, worry, and/or panic. The effects of anxiety disorders include disrupted sleep, difficulty concentrating, and somatic complaints.

Current treatment
Antidepressant and antianxiety medication are frequently used to treat depression and anxiety, often in conjunction with psychotherapy. However, medication side

Table 1
Effects of tai chi on psychological, physical, or physiologic systems

Psychological, Physical, or Physiologic Systems	Tai Chi Component	Proposed Mechanism of Action
Brain health and cognitive decline	Aerobic exercise	• Endorphin release • Mood stabilization • Neurocognitive changes, including angiogenesis and neurogenesis
	Expectation and intention	• Improved self-perception, including self-efficacy and self-esteem
	Memorization and sequencing of poses	• Synaptogenesis
	Mindfulness and meditation	• Relaxation • Stress reduction
Mental health: depression and anxiety	Imagery	• Focused attention • Increased parasympathetic nervous system activity
	Flexibility/range of motion	• Improved coordination • Improved sense of well-being and mood
	Intentional movement	• Improved coordination • Reduced fear of falling
	Meditative breathing	• Alterations in stress-response pathways: decreased sympathetic system activity and increased parasympathetic nervous system activity • Decreased somatic symptoms
	Mindfulness	• Relaxation • Stress reduction
	Social support	• Increased self-efficacy and self-esteem
Sleep	Mindfulness and focus	• Relaxation • Stress reduction
	Meditative breathing	• Decreased sympathetic nervous system activity • Stress reduction
	Gentle physical motion	• Increased extremity/joint strength and flexibility • Reduced musculoskeletal pain (such as from joint pain)

Cardiovascular: heart failure	Aerobic exercise	• Improved exercise tolerance caused by/because of increased cardiac output and oxygenation of blood
	Correct body posture	• Reveals an individual's internal sense of well-being/mood
	Meditative breathing	• Alterations in stress-response pathways: decreased sympathetic system activity and increased parasympathetic nervous system activity
		• Decreased somatic symptoms
	Mindfulness	• Awareness of moment-to-moment sensations trains the individual to hold attention/mental focus
Cardiovascular: stroke	Aerobic exercise	• Neurocognitive changes, including angiogenesis and neurogenesis
	Correct body posture	• Reveals an individual's internal sense of well-being and mood
	Imagery and visualization	• Mental practice that involves repetitive cognitive rehearsal of physical movements
	Mindfulness	• Awareness of moment-to-moment sensations trains the individual to hold attention and mental focus
Fall prevention: balance and mobility	Flexibility	• Dynamic stretching during movements
	Muscle strengthening	• Slightly flexed stances load leg muscles and bones
	Structural integration	• Correct body posture and alignment
	Weight shifting	• Postural control and stability

effects and lack of efficacy have stimulated research to supplement or reduce reliance on its use.[16] Tai chi has been studied as a complement to both antidepressant medication and psychotherapy, with positive results in adults of all ages, in pregnancy, and among people with chronic illnesses.[17]

Tai chi intervention studies
A systematic review and meta-analysis examined 40 studies, including randomized and nonrandomized trials studying the effectiveness of tai chi on multiple psychological health outcomes.[18] Intervention groups were compared with control groups consisting of health education, usual daily activity/routine medication, and waitlist. The findings indicate an association between tai chi and decreased depression and anxiety and improved self-perception, including self-efficacy and self-esteem.

Measures
Outcomes measured included self-reported depression and anxiety (Beck Depression Inventory, Center for Epidemiologic Studies Depression Scale [CES-D],[19] Profile of Mood States and subscales),[20] self-esteem (Rosenberg Self-esteem Scale),[21] overall health status, QOL, and physiologic markers of stress (eg, cortisol and C-reactive protein levels).

Proposed therapeutic effects
Several mechanisms of tai chi exercise may contribute to psychological benefits, including the association between exercise and psychological health; meditation's positive effect on mood, stress and affect; and the benefits of social support (see **Table 1**). Because of its beneficial multiple components, tai chi exercise is a promising strategy to supplement conventional therapies for depression and anxiety, and to enhance overall psychological well-being.

Sleep

Problem/cause
Good-quality sleep is restorative to the mind and body, with benefits including improved mental, physical, and immune function. However, approximately 1 in 3 American adults do not get the recommended 7 to 8 hours of sleep per day.[22] Reasons for poor sleep include lifestyle behaviors and medical conditions such as cardiopulmonary disorders, pain, or anxiety.

Current treatment
Pharmacologic treatment of sleep disorders, whether over-the-counter or prescription medications, are associated with side effects such as lightheadedness, prolonged drowsiness, and memory issues. Nonpharmacologic strategies to improve sleep quality include cognitive behavior therapy as well as behavior modifications, referred to as sleep hygiene, and include maintaining routine sleep patterns; avoiding large meals, caffeine, and alcoholic drinks; and restricting strenuous exercise before bedtime.[22,23]

Tai chi intervention studies
In addition to pharmacologic and behavioral interventions, the effect of tai chi exercise on sleep quality and daytime sleepiness has been studied in several populations, including community-dwelling adults, older adults, and adults with chronic health conditions.[24] Systematic reviews and meta-analyses lend support to the benefit of tai chi for improved sleep. Most reviews have focused on adults and older adults (mean age range, 21–77 years old) and included people with both moderate sleep complaints and those with clinical diagnoses of insomnia.[25–27] Several studies specifically focused on patients with chronic conditions, including fibromyalgia and cardiovascular or

cerebrovascular conditions. The tai chi intervention participants were compared with control groups assigned to health education, low-impact exercise, waitlist, and usual care. Interventions ranged from 8 weeks to 24 weeks, with varying frequencies, the most common tai chi intervention being 3 times per week.

Measures

Sleep scales included the Pittsburgh Sleep Quality Index[28] and the Epworth Sleepiness Scale[29] measuring time to sleep, length of sleep time, feelings on awakening, daytime sleepiness, and overall QOL.[24,26,30–32] For study participants with fibromyalgia and cardiovascular or cerebrovascular conditions, additional measures collected included condition-specific and disease-specific symptom reporting, such as the Fibromyalgia Improvement Questionnaire,[33] and, for patients with heart failure (HF), the Minnesota Living with Health Failure Questionnaire (MLHFQ).[34] Measures of depression, functional status, physical performance, pain, self-efficacy, and QOL were also assessed.

Proposed therapeutic effects

Several of tai chi exercise's components are proposed to improve sleep quality, including psychological benefits of mindfulness and physical benefits from tai chi's gentle movements (see **Table 1**). Tai chi stimulates the parasympathetic nervous system, inducing calmness from the meditative aspects, reduces stress, and has a positive impact on self-esteem.[18] For chronic health conditions affecting sleep (eg, osteoarthritis), tai chi improves joint range of motion and musculoskeletal strength and stability, thereby decreasing joint pain and contributing to improved sleep through interruption of the pain cycle.[35] There is strong evidence to support tai chi as a strategy to improve and enhance sleep quality in healthy community-dwelling adults and those with chronic health conditions. As stated by Raman and colleagues,[26] "As is the essence of many behavioral therapies, Tai Chi may have profound salutogenic effects on improving sleep quality, and these effects come only with consistent practice."

CARDIOVASCULAR HEALTH: HEART FAILURE
Problem/Cause

Approximately 26 million people worldwide have HF, with the prevalence of HF increasing because of an aging population, and better management of the condition.[36,37] In the United States, an estimated 6.2 million adults have HF, whereas the incidence of HF is estimated to affect 21 in 1000 adults 65 years of age and older. HF prevalence is expected to increase to 8 million adults by the year 2030, with direct costs in the United States expected to reach $69.8 billion.[38] Adults with HF frequently report poor exercise tolerance, reduced QOL, depression, and recurrent hospitalizations.[39,40]

Current Treatment

Guidelines from the American College of Cardiology/American Heart Association (AHA) task force for the management of HF provide recommendations for pharmacologic treatment of HF with reduced ejection fraction (HFrEF; <45%) or those with HF with preserved ejection fraction (HFpEF; ≥45%), along with management of important comorbidities.[37] In addition, these guidelines recommend assessment of B-type natriuretic peptide (BNP) or N-terminal pro-BNP (NT-proBNP) to establish severity of HF. The European Society of Cardiology HF guidelines also recommend that adults with HF participate in regular exercise to improve aerobic capacity and QOL.[41] A recent systematic review and meta-analysis found that exercise-based cardiac rehabilitation for adults with HFrEF or HFpEF was effective in reducing overall hospitalizations and improving QOL.[39] However, cardiac rehabilitation services for HF are greatly underused, with only 10% of patients receiving a referral when discharged from the hospital.[42,43]

Tai Chi Intervention Studies

A recent systematic review and meta-analysis of clinical trials published between 2004 and 2019 examined the benefits of tai chi among adults with HF.[44] The findings indicate that adults with HF in the tai chi group had significantly better exercise capacity, improved QOL, less depression, and lower BNP levels after the intervention, compared with controls.[44]

Measures

Among adults with HF, the 6-minute walk test[45] is frequently used as an indicator of exercise capacity, whereas the MLHFQ[34] is commonly used among adults with HF to assess QOL. Depression can be assessed using a variety of measures, including the CES-D,[19] the Patient Health Questionnaire,[46] or the Patient-reported Outcomes Measurement Information System (PROMIS)–Depression[47] scales. Blood tests for biomarkers (ie, BNP or NT-proBNP) are used to assess HF severity. According to the European Society of Cardiology (ESC) HF guidelines, blood test values for BNP greater than 100 pg/mL or NT-proBNP greater than 300 pg/mL indicate symptomatic HF, warranting further diagnostic investigation.[41]

Proposed Therapeutic Effects

Improvements in physical health (ie, exercise capacity, BNP levels) following a tai chi intervention likely stem from an increase in cardiac output and an enhancement of the innate ability of muscles to extract and use oxygen from the blood.[48] Improvements in mental health (ie, QOL and depression) often coincide with better physical health. It is well known that tai chi fosters balanced, open, and relaxed postures through proper body alignment. Recent research reports that correct body posture plays a key role in helping individuals recover from depression[49] (see **Table 1**).

CARDIOVASCULAR HEALTH: STROKE
Problem/Cause

According to the World Stroke Organization, worldwide roughly 14 million people experience a stroke each year.[50] In the United States, nearly 800,000 people have a stroke each year. There are currently 7 million adults living in the United States who are stroke survivors. The main risk factors for stroke include hypertension, atrial fibrillation, smoking, diabetes, high cholesterol level, poor diet, and physical inactivity.[38] Stroke is a leading cause of long-term disability among survivors.[38]

Current Treatment

Stroke rehabilitation and recovery guidelines[51] underscore the need for a multidisciplinary team working in conjunction with the stroke survivor, their family and friends, or caregivers to maximize rehabilitation effectiveness, to achieve optimal outcomes. In the past, stroke rehabilitation (ie, physical, occupational, and/or speech) occurs during the first 3 to 4 months following a stroke, to prevent falls, improve mobility and activities of daily living (ADLs), and reduce disability and depressive symptoms.[51] In addition, stroke rehabilitation includes assessments in communication/speech, cognitive function, and sensory impairments, to tailor individual rehabilitation and recovery needs.[51] Recent research studies indicate that physical activity and/or longer rehabilitation is beneficial for stroke survivors, even several years after they had their strokes.[51,52] The AHA/American Stroke Association (ASA) recommends regular physical activity/exercise for stroke survivors, because it has been shown to improve physical function, assist with ADLs, increase QOL, and reduce the risk for subsequent cardiovascular events.[53]

Tai Chi Intervention Studies

Prior systematic reviews and meta-analyses examining the benefits of tai chi among stroke survivors have primarily focused on physical function, reporting significant improvements in balance, gait, and ADLs.[54–56] Limited research has examined psychosocial benefits of a tai chi intervention among stroke survivors, compared with controls.[32,57,58] One small randomized clinical trial reported better QOL and sleep quality, with less depression and anxiety among stroke survivors after 12-weeks of tai chi (1 hour, once per week), compared with traditional rehabilitation.[57]

Measures

Physical function after stroke is typically assessed using standard measures, such as the modified Rankin Scale, Functional Independence Measure, Barthel Index of Activities of Daily Living, and/or Berg Balance Scale.[59] QOL measures typically include Medical Outcomes Study Short Form 36 (SF-36) or the Stroke Specific Quality of Life Scale.[59] To assess cognitive function, the MMSE or the Montreal Cognitive Assessment are used.[59] The Hospital Anxiety and Depression Scale,[59] CES-D,[19] and Neuro-QOL (QOL in Neurological Disorders) Depression and Anxiety Short Forms can be used to assess poststroke symptoms.[60] Several outcomes measures with good psychometric properties appropriate for use among stroke survivors can be obtained free of charge at HealthMeasures (http://www.healthmeasures.net/). HealthMeasures is the official information and distribution center for PROMIS, Neuro-QoL, NIH Toolbox, and ASCQ-Me (Adult Sickle Cell QOL Measurement Information System), which were developed and evaluated with National Institutes of Health (NIH) funding.

Proposed Therapeutic Effects

During tai chi practice, imagery and visualization, sometimes referred to as mental practice, are used to guide an individual toward certain kinesthetic, emotion, and energetic states (eg, individuals are instructed to wave hands like clouds).[61] Research has shown that the brain is able to respond to repetitive, learning-based strategies even several years after a stroke.[62] Mental practice involves repetitive cognitive rehearsal of physical movements in the absence of physical ability, such as occurs among stroke survivors with hemiparesis. Moreover, the same neural and muscular areas of the body are activated during mental practice as during physical practice of the same skill. However, mental practice is most effective when combined with physical practice, which occurs while practicing tai chi.[62] During tai chi practice, individuals interact with the instructor and other students, which fosters social support. For stroke survivors with depression, these group-based tai chi classes can create a sense of belonging, leading to fewer depressive symptoms[63–65] (see **Table 1**).

FALL PREVENTION: BALANCE AND MOBILITY
Problem/Cause

Every 19 minutes, an older adult dies from a fall; every 11 seconds an older adult is treated in an emergency room for a fall-related injury.[66] In 2017, unintentional falls were the leading cause of injury deaths among adults 65 years of age and older living in the United States.[67] Among older adults, slow gait speeds (<0.6 m/s) increase fall risk (poor balance/postural control) and are associated with the fear of falling.[68–70]

Current Treatment

The CDC's Stopping Elderly Accidents, Deaths, and Injuries (STEADI) program was developed as a multifactorial approach to fall prevention consisting of 3 core elements: screening for fall risk, assessing for modifiable risk factors, and prescribing evidence-based interventions to reduce fall risk.[71,72] Screening of all adults aged 65 years and older is recommended annually, asking 3 questions: (1) have you fallen in the past year, (2) do you feel unsteady when standing or walking, and (3) do you worry about falling? The STEADI Web site contains materials for both providers and patients to assess and intervene to reduce fall risk, all of which are open access and free of charge (https://www.cdc.gov/steadi/). There several evidence-based fall prevention programs for community-dwelling older adults, including A Matter of Balance, Otago Exercise Program, Stay Active and Independent for Life, and Tai Ji Quan: Moving for Better Balance.[5,73]

Tai Chi Intervention Studies

Several systematic reviews and meta-analyses have been conducted in the past 10 years, examining the effectiveness of tai chi to reduce falls/fall risk, and improve balance and gait/mobility.[55,74–77] Empirical evidence indicates that tai chi significantly reduces fall incidence among adults with a risk of falling,[74] and leads to better balance and mobility among community-dwelling adults, even those with chronic health conditions.[55,75,78] Moreover, community-based implementation of a tai chi program among older adults (N = 511, mean age = 75 years) across numerous senior centers (N = 32) led to a 49% reduction in the number of falls.[79]

Measures

The Timed Up and Go (TUG)[80] test is commonly used to determine fall risk. The TUG measures the time taken for a person to rise from an arm chair, walk 3 m (may use assistive devices), turn, walk back to chair, and sit down. A TUG greater than or equal to 12 seconds is used as a cutoff for high fall risk among community-dwelling older adults.[81] The 4-Stage Balance Test[82] assess 4 standing positions that get progressively harder to maintain (ie, parallel, semitandem, tandem, and stand on 1 foot). Adults unable to hold the tandem stand for at least 10 seconds are at increased risk of falling, needing a referral for balance exercises. Gait is commonly assessed using a 4-m gait speed test, and is reported as meters per second.[83,84] Leg strength, which is integral to prevention of falls, can be assessed using a chair stand test.[83,84] This test measures the time that is needed to perform 5 rises from a chair to an upright position as fast as possible without use of the arms.[83]

Proposed Therapeutic Effects

Tai chi integrates motor, sensory, and cognitive components to improve balance, strength, and gait, leading to fewer falls.[79,85] It is well established that the integrated movements of tai chi result in less strain, greater power with less effort, and better balance. The slow movements and shifting of body weight to 1 leg improve balance. Slightly flexed stances load leg muscles and bones, leading to better strength, with flexibility enhanced through dynamic stretching because of the slow, relaxed, repetitive movements during tai chi practice[75,86] (see **Table 1**).

SUMMARY

Tai chi has grown in popularity and accessibility over the past 2 decades. Scientific evidence continues to advance the understanding of tai chi's multifaceted health benefits, including positive effects on cognition, depression, anxiety, sleep, cardiovascular health, and fall prevention. Nurses interact with patients across the lifespan both for health maintenance and disease management and can assist patients to seek qualified tai chi instructors or to explore tai chi classes appropriate for their patients' needs. Through this ancient form of exercise, nurses can promote health and well-being in physical, mental, emotional, and social domains.

DISCLOSURE

The authors have nothing to disclose.

REFERENCES

1. World Health Organization. WHOQOL: Measuring Quality of Life. 2020. Available at: https://www.who.int/healthinfo/survey/whoqol-qualityoflife/en/. Accessed April 4, 2020.
2. Office of Disease Prevention and Health Promotion. Healthy People. 2020. Available at: https://www.healthypeople.gov/. Accessed April 22, 2020.
3. Lauche R, Wayne PM, Dobos G, et al. Prevalence, patterns, and predictors of T'ai Chi and Qigong use in the United States: results of a nationally representative survey. J Altern Complement Med 2016;22(4):336–42.
4. Cui H, Wang Q, Pedersen M, et al. The safety of tai chi: a meta-analysis of adverse events in randomized controlled trials. Contemp Clin Trials 2019;82: 85–92.
5. Stevens JA, Burns ER. CDC Compendium of effective fall interventions: what works for community-dwelling older adults. 3rd ed. Atlanta (GA): Division of Unintentional Injury Prevention, National Center for Injury Prevention and Control, Centers for Disease Control and Prevention; 2015.
6. National Center for Complementary and Integrative Health. Tai Chi and Qi Gong: In Depth. 2020. Available at: https://www.nccih.nih.gov/health/tai-chi-and-qi-gong-in-depth. Accessed April 22, 2020.
7. Centers for Disease Control and Prevention. Healthy Brain Initiative. 2020. Available at: http://www.cdc.gov/aging/healthybrain/index.htm. Accessed April 4, 2020.
8. Voss MW, Nagamatsu LS, Liu-Ambrose T, et al. Exercise, brain, and cognition across the life span. J Appl Physiol 2011;111(5):1505–13.
9. Ainsworth BE, Haskell WL, Herrmann SD, et al. 2011 Compendium of Physical Activities: a second update of codes and MET values. Med Sci Sports Exerc 2011;43(8):1575–81.
10. Centers for Disease Control and Prevention. Physical Activity: Recommendations & Guidelines. 2020. https://www.cdc.gov/physicalactivity/resources/recommendations. html. Accessed April 4, 2020.
11. Wayne PM, Walsh JN, Taylor-Piliae RE, et al. Effect of Tai Chi on cognitive performance in older adults: Systematic review and meta-analysis. J Am Geriatr Soc 2014;62(1):25–39.
12. Folstein MF, Folstein SE, McHugh PR. "Mini-mental state": A practical method for grading the cognitive state of patients for the clinician. J Psychiatr Res 1975; 12(3):189–98.

13. Strauss E, Sherman EMS, Spreen O. A compendium of neuropsychological tests: administration, tests, norms, and commentary. 3rd edition. New York: Oxford University Press; 2006.
14. Office of Disease Prevention and Health Promotion. Health-Related Quality of Life & Well-Being. 2020. Available at: https://www.healthypeople.gov/2020/topics-objectives/topic/health-related-quality-of-life-well-being. Accessed April 22, 2020.
15. Centers for Disease Control and Prevention. Depression. 2020. Available at: https://www.cdc.gov/nchs/fastats/depression.htm. Accessed April 4, 2020.
16. Centers for Disease Control and Prevention. Mental Health Conditions: Depression and Anxiety. 2015. Available at: https://www.cdc.gov/tobacco/campaign/tips/diseases/depression-anxiety.html. Accessed April 4, 2020.
17. National Center for Complementary and Integrative Health. Relaxation Techniques for Health. 2016. Available at: https://www.nccih.nih.gov/health/relaxation-techniques-for-health. Accessed April 4, 2020.
18. Wang C, Bannuru R, Ramel J, et al. Tai Chi on psychological well-being: systematic review and meta-analysis. BMC Complement Altern Med 2010;10(1):23.
19. Radloff LS. The CES-D Scale: A self report depression scale for research in the general population. Appl Psychol Meas 1977;1(3):385–401.
20. McNair DM. Profile of mood states. San Diego (CA): Educational and industrial testing service; 1992.
21. Rosenberg M. Conceiving the Self. New York: Basic Books; 1979.
22. Centers for Disease Control and Prevention. Sleep and Sleep Disorders. 2020. Available at: https://www.cdc.gov/sleep/index.html. Accessed April 22, 2020.
23. American Academy of Sleep Medicine. Sleep Education. 2020. Available at: http://sleepeducation.org/essentials-in-sleep/healthy-sleep-habits. Accessed April 4, 2020.
24. Irwin MR, Olmstead R, Motivala SJ. Improving sleep quality in older adults with moderate sleep complaints: A randomized controlled trial of Tai Chi Chih. Sleep 2008;31(7):1001–8.
25. Cheng CA, Chiu YW, Wu D, et al. Effectiveness of Tai Chi on fibromyalgia patients: A meta-analysis of randomized controlled trials. Complement Ther Med 2019; 46:1–8.
26. Raman G, Zhang Y, Minichiello VJ, et al. Tai Chi improves sleep quality in healthy adults and patients with chronic conditions: A systematic review and meta-analysis. J Sleep Disord Ther 2013;2(6).
27. Wang F, Eun-Kyoung Lee O, Feng F, et al. The effect of meditative movement on sleep quality: A systematic review. Sleep Med Rev 2016;30:43–52.
28. Buysse DJ, Reynolds CF 3rd, Monk TH, et al. The Pittsburgh Sleep Quality Index: a new instrument for psychiatric practice and research. Psychiatry Res 1989; 28(2):193–213.
29. The Epworth Sleepiness Scale. 2020. Available at: https://epworthsleepinessscale.com/about-the-ess/. Accessed April 4, 2020.
30. Du S, Dong J, Zhang H, et al. Taichi exercise for self-rated sleep quality in older people: A systematic review and meta-analysis. Int J Nurs Stud 2015;52(1): 368–79.
31. Li F, Fisher KJ, Harmer P, et al. Tai chi and self-rated quality of sleep and daytime sleepiness in older adults: a randomized controlled trial. J Am Geriatr Soc 2004; 52(6):892–900.
32. Taylor-Piliae RE, Hoke TM, Hepworth JT, et al. Effect of Tai Chi on physical function, fall rates and quality of life among older stroke survivors. Arch Phys Med Rehabil 2014;95(5):816–24.

33. American College of Rheumatology. Fibromyalgia Impact Questionnaire (FIQ). 2020. Available at: https://www.rheumatology.org/I-Am-A/Rheumatologist/Research/Clinician-Researchers/Fibromyalgia-Impact-Questionnaire-FIQ. Accessed April 4, 20.

34. Rector TS, Kubo SH, Cohn JN. Patients' self-assessment of their congestive heart failure: Content, reliability and validity of a new measure, the Minnesota Living With Heart Failure Questionnaire. Heart Fail 1987;3:198–209.

35. Wang C, Schmid CH, Hibberd PL, et al. Tai Chi is effective in treating knee osteoarthritis: a randomized controlled trial. Arthritis Rheum 2009;61(11):1545–53.

36. Savarese G, Lund LH. Global public health burden of heart failure. Card Fail Rev 2017;3(1):7–11.

37. Yancy CW, Jessup M, Bozkurt B, et al. 2017 ACC/AHA/HFSA Focused update of the 2013 ACCF/AHA guideline for the management of heart failure: A report of the American College of Cardiology/American Heart Association Task Force on Clinical Practice Guidelines and the Heart Failure Society of America. Circulation 2017;136(6):e137–61.

38. Benjamin EJ, Muntner P, Alonso A, et al. Heart disease and stroke statistics-2019 update: A report from the American Heart Association. Circulation 2019;139(10):e56–528.

39. Long L, Mordi IR, Bridges C, et al. Exercise-based cardiac rehabilitation for adults with heart failure. Cochrane Database Syst Rev 2019;(1):CD003331.

40. Schopfer DW, Forman DE. Growing relevance of cardiac rehabilitation for an older population with heart failure. J Card Fail 2016;22(12):1015–22.

41. Ponikowski P, Voors AA, Anker SD, et al. 2016 ESC Guidelines for the diagnosis and treatment of acute and chronic heart failure: The task force for the diagnosis and treatment of acute and chronic heart failure of the European Society of Cardiology (ESC). Developed with the special contribution of the Heart Failure Association (HFA) of the ESC. Eur J Heart Fail 2016;18(8):891–975.

42. Golwala H, Pandey A, Ju C, et al. Temporal trends and factors associated with cardiac rehabilitation referral among patients hospitalized with heart failure: Findings from get with the guidelines-heart failure registry. J Am Coll Cardiol 2015;66(8):917–26.

43. Forman DE, Sanderson BK, Josephson RA, et al. American college of cardiology's prevention of cardiovascular diseases. Heart failure as a newly approved diagnosis for cardiac rehabilitation: Challenges and opportunities. J Am Coll Cardiol 2015;65(24):2652–9.

44. Taylor-Piliae RE, Finley BA. Benefits of Tai Chi exercise among adults with chronic heart failure: A systematic review and meta-Analysis. J Cardiovasc Nurs 2020. https://doi.org/10.1097/JCN.0000000000000703 [Online ahead of print].

45. Guazzi M, Dickstein K, Vicenzi M, et al. Six-minute walk test and cardiopulmonary exercise testing in patients with chronic heart failure: a comparative analysis on clinical and prognostic insights. Circ Heart Fail 2009;2(6):549–55.

46. Kroenke K, Spitzer RL, Williams JB. The PHQ-9: validity of a brief depression severity measure. J Gen Intern Med 2001;16(9):606–13.

47. Pilkonis PA, Choi SW, Reise SP, et al. Item banks for measuring emotional distress from the Patient-Reported Outcomes Measurement Information System (PROMIS(R)): Depression, anxiety, and anger. Assessment 2011;18(3):263–83.

48. Cattadori G, Segurini C, Picozzi A, et al. Exercise and heart failure: an update. ESC Heart Fail 2018;5(2):222–32.

49. Veenstra L, Schneider IK, Koole SL. Embodied mood regulation: the impact of body posture on mood recovery, negative thoughts, and mood-congruent recall. Cogn Emot 2017;31(7):1361–76.
50. World Stroke Organization. Global Stroke Fact Sheet. 2019. Available at: www.world-stroke.org. Accessed April 4, 2020.
51. Winstein CJ, Stein J, Arena R, et al. Guidelines for adult stroke rehabilitation and recovery: A guideline for healthcare professionals from the American Heart Association/American Stroke Association. Stroke 2016;47(6):e98–169.
52. Korner-Bitensky N. When does stroke rehabilitation end? Int J Stroke 2013; 8(1):8–10.
53. Billinger SA, Arena R, Bernhardt J, et al. Physical activity and exercise recommendations for stroke survivors: a statement for healthcare professionals from the American Heart Association/American Stroke Association. Stroke 2014; 45(8):2532–53.
54. Wu S, Chen J, Wang S, et al. Effect of Tai Chi Exercise on balance function of stroke patients: A meta-analysis. Med Sci Monit Basic Res 2018;24:210–5.
55. Li GY, Wang W, Liu GL, et al. Effects of Tai Chi on balance and gait in stroke survivors: A systematic meta-analysis of randomized controlled trials. J Rehabil Med 2018;50(7):582–8.
56. Lyu D, Lyu X, Zhang Y, et al. Tai Chi for Stroke Rehabilitation: A systematic review and meta-analysis of randomized controlled trials. Front Physiol 2018;9:983.
57. Wang W, Sawada M, Noriyama Y, et al. Tai Chi exercise versus rehabilitation for the elderly with cerebral vascular disorder: a single-blinded randomized controlled trial. Psychogeriatrics 2010;10(3):160–6.
58. Hwang I, Song R, Ahn S, et al. Exploring the adaptability of Tai Chi to stroke rehabilitation. Rehabil Nurs 2019;44(4):221–9.
59. Salter K, Campbell N, Richardson M, et al. Chapter 20: Outcome measures in stroke rehabilitation. In: Evidence-based review of stroke rehabilitation. Ontario (Canada): 2018. Available at: http://www.ebrsr.com//evidence-review.
60. National Institute of Neurological Disorders and Stroke. User manual for the quality of life in neurological disorders (Neuro-QoL) measures, version 2.0. National Institute of Neurological Disorders and Stroke; 2015. Available at: https://www.healthmeasures.net/explore-measurement-systems/neuro-qol.
61. Robins JL, Elswick RK, McCain NL. The story of the evolution of a unique tai chi form: origins, philosophy, and research. J Holist Nurs 2012;30(3):134–46.
62. Page SJ, Peters H. Mental practice: applying motor PRACTICE and neuroplasticity principles to increase upper extremity function. Stroke 2014;45(11):3454–60.
63. Taylor-Piliae RE, Coull BM. Poor quality of life and low social support are predictive of depressive symptoms in chronic stroke. Stroke 2012;43(2; Suppl 1). Abstract 2351.
64. Yeh GY, Chan CW, Wayne PM, et al. The impact of tai chi exercise on self-efficacy, social support, and empowerment in heart failure: insights from a qualitative substudy from a randomized controlled trial. PLoS One 2016;11(5):e0154678.
65. Ma C, Zhou W, Tang Q, et al. The impact of group-based Tai Chi on health-status outcomes among community-dwelling older adults with hypertension. Heart Lung 2018;47(4):337–44.
66. National Council on Aging. Falls prevention: fact sheet. Available at: https://www.ncoa.org/resources/falls-prevention-fact-sheet/2018. Accessed April 4, 2020.
67. Kochanek KD, Murphy SL, Xu JQ, et al. Deaths: final data for 2017. In: Reports: National Vital Statistics. Hyattsville (MD): National Center for Health Statistics; 2019.

68. Verghese J, Holtzer R, Lipton RB, et al. Quantitative gait markers and incident fall risk in older adults. J Gerontol A Biol Sci Med Sci 2009;64(8):896–901.
69. Studenski S, Perera S, Patel K, et al. Gait speed and survival in older adults. JAMA 2011;305(1):50–8.
70. Abellan van Kan G, Rolland Y, Andrieu S, et al. Gait speed at usual pace as a predictor of adverse outcomes in community-dwelling older people an International Academy on Nutrition and Aging (IANA) Task Force. J Nutr Health Aging 2009;13(10):881–9.
71. Stevens JA, Smith ML, Parker EM, et al. Implementing a clinically based fall prevention program. Am J Lifestyle Med 2020;14(1):71–7.
72. Stevens JA, Phelan EA. Development of STEADI: a fall prevention resource for health care providers. Health Promot Pract 2013;14(5):706–14.
73. Taylor-Piliae RE, Peterson R, Mohler MJ. Clinical and community strategies to prevent falls and fall-related injuries among community-dwelling older adults. Nurs Clin North Am 2017;52(3):489–97.
74. Lomas-Vega R, Obrero-Gaitan E, Molina-Ortega FJ, et al. Tai Chi for risk of falls: A meta-analysis. J Am Geriatr Soc 2017;65(9):2037–43.
75. Huang Y, Liu X. Improvement of balance control ability and flexibility in the elderly Tai Chi Chuan (TCC) practitioners: a systematic review and meta-analysis. Arch Gerontol Geriatr 2015;60(2):233–8.
76. Liu H, Frank A. Tai chi as a balance improvement exercise for older adults: a systematic review. J Geriatr Phys Ther 2010;33(3):103–9.
77. Taylor E, Taylor-Piliae RE. The effects of Tai Chi on physical and psychosocial function among persons with multiple sclerosis: A systematic review. Complement Ther Med 2017;31:100–8.
78. Hackney ME, Wolf SL. Impact of Tai Chi Chu'an practice on balance and mobility in older adults: an integrative review of 20 years of research. J Geriatr Phys Ther 2014;37(3):127–35.
79. Li F, Harmer P, Fitzgerald K. Implementing an evidence-based fall prevention intervention in community senior centers. Am J Public Health 2016;106(11): 2026–31.
80. Podsiadlo D, Richardson S. The timed "Up & Go": A test of basic functional mobility for frail elderly persons. J Am Geriatr Soc 1991;39(2):142–8.
81. Bischoff HA, Stahelin HB, Monsch AU, et al. Identifying a cut-off point for normal mobility: a comparison of the timed 'up and go' test in community-dwelling and institutionalised elderly women. Age Ageing 2003;32(3):315–20.
82. Rossiter-Fornoff JE, Wolf SL, Wolfson LI, et al. A cross-sectional validation study of the FICSIT common data base static balance measures. Frailty and Injuries: Cooperative Studies of Intervention Techniques. J Gerontol A Biol Sci Med Sci 1995;50(6):M291–7.
83. Guralnik JM, Simonsick EM, Ferrucci L, et al. A short physical performance battery assessing lower extremity function: association with self-reported disability and prediction of mortality and nursing home admission. J Gerontol 1994; 49(2):M85–94.
84. Taylor-Piliae RE, Latt LD, Hepworth JT, et al. Predictors of gait velocity among community-dwelling stroke survivors. Gait Posture 2012;35(3):395–9.
85. Li F. Transforming traditional Tai Ji Quan techniques into integrative movement therapy–Tai Ji Quan: Moving for Better Balance. J Sport Health Sci 2014; 3(1):9–15.

86. Taylor-Piliae RE, Haskell WL, Stotts NA, et al. Improvement in balance, strength, and flexibility after 12 weeks of Tai chi exercise in ethnic Chinese adults with cardiovascular disease risk factors. Altern Ther Health Med 2006;12(2):50–8.
87. Yang Y, Grubisch SA. Taijiquan: the art of nurturing, the science of power. Champaign (IL): Zhenwu Publications; 2005.
88. Jun Y, Tom R, Repetto B, et al. Yang family Tai Chi essentials. Bothell (WA): International Yang Family Tai Chi Chuan Association; 2020.
89. Eldh AC, Ekman I, Ehnfors M. Conditions for patient participation and nonparticipation in health care. Nurs Ethics 2006;13(5):503–14.

APPENDIX 1: ADVISING PATIENTS INTERESTED IN TAI CHI EXERCISE: A TAI CHI TEACHER'S PERSPECTIVE

Commonality between styles

There are 6 major tai chi family styles: Chen, Yang, Wu Hao, Wu, Sun, and He. Although each style has its unique characteristics and style, they share some similar tai chi traditions.[87]

Overarching Purpose

Despite the martial art origins of tai chi, health preservation and self-cultivation have become the emphasis of current practice.[88] Health preservation involves bringing systemic harmony and developing psychophysical strength and stamina. Self-cultivation pertains to the nurturing process of mind, body, and spirit.

Philosophy

Tai chi is founded on traditional Chinese medicine's perspective of meridians and 5-elements theory of fire, water, wood, metal, and earth.[88] Optimal health is achievable by maintaining equilibrium and understanding of the correlative relationship between the pathways, internal organs, and physical body. In tai chi practice, these concepts help to explain (1) the dynamic and ever-evolving yin and yang states; and (2) the connection and centering of emotions, internal organs, and the 5 tai chi positions (forward, back, left, right, and center) and directions (east, south, west, north, and center).

Principles

Across styles, tai chi principles are crucial in guiding skill refinement and optimizing health benefits.[88] Their interconnectivity and coexistence in each movement make tai chi practice captivating, reflective, meditative, and intriguing. The following are some commonly shared principles among the major tai chi styles:

- Intention. Every movement begins with an intent, which is heart centered. Heart-centeredness promotes self-cultivation of the inner spirt, and at a deeper level of practice can influence one's world view.[87] Intention gives rise to qi, energy, which in turn supports the subsequent movement. This process contrasts with the practice of traditional martial arts in exerting force and physical strength.

- Relaxed state. Song, or relaxed, in tai chi consists of 2 interwoven components. It pertains to maintaining mental calmness, focused attention, and alertness to bring about the continuous physical state of relaxing and lengthening the joints and tendons. It embeds the duo quality of soft and hard, whereby inner strength emerges from the relaxed state to generate flexibility and yielding in motion like a whip. Maintaining this state in tai chi practice is crucial to optimize health benefits.

- Alignment. Visualizing a gentle lifting or upward-reaching sensation on the crown of the head and relaxing the spine facilitates natural alignment.

- Breathing. Tai chi places minimal emphasis on how to breathe but focuses on movement intent and its coordinated natural abdominal breathing. Breathing is quiet, smooth, and deep, with a fully relaxed upper chest and shoulder complex.

- Movement. Every step, turn, kick, push, and punch is performed precisely and slowly for internal and external integration and for proper weight distribution in the leading and supporting legs. In all tai chi styles, waist and hip flexors, or kua, direct trunk movements, which in turn generates arm movements. The resultant series of movements are connected, coordinated, fluid, light, and effortless.

- Unified mind and body. Coordinated movements necessitate the integration of mental alertness, light upper body, flexible waist and hip flexors, and firm grounding of the feet.

- Mindset. The heart-mind–directed tai chi practice emphasizes adherence to the principles, attention to details, persistence in practice, openness to growth, and adaptability to change.

Assisting patients to select a teacher

Like any subject matter teacher, tai chi teachers play a significant role in facilitating learning and optimizing health benefits. Careful selection of a tai chi teacher with the advocacy of a nurse increases the prospect of patient participation and of attaining patients' health and wellness goals.[89] Following are some suggested steps for nurses to assist patients with selecting a tai chi teacher.

Know What the Patient Wants

It is important to know why the patient is taking a class or whether 1-on-1 sessions would be appropriate, because this determines the type of class and teaching that can best achieve the patient's goals.

Be Cognizant of the Patient's Commitment Level

If the patient is curious about tai chi and wants to try it for several weeks, any teacher would likely serve this need. However, if the patient has chronic pain or arthritis, or is recovering from surgery, much effort and commitment is necessary. The process could revolve around gradual adjustment phases, such as increasing body awareness of compensatory movements and relearning natural movement patterns, coordination, and alignment.

Consider Participation Options

Tai chi group classes are often available as drop-in or skill-based classes. Drop-in classes are most suitable for beginners or those who want gentle movements to complement their other activities. Skill-based classes are generally divided into levels and are suitable for those who plan to build their tai chi skills long term, according to their readiness and time commitment. Some teachers offer 1-on-1 sessions, which are particularly useful for patients who want to focus on specific tai chi skills for their personal interests or to address specific physical needs such as chronic pain or fall prevention.

Advise the Patient to Meet with the Teacher

At present, no standardized tai chi teaching certification is available in the United States. Teachers have great latitude in how and what they teach. This latitude makes understanding the teacher's teaching philosophy and methods crucial, especially when recommending tai chi to patients. Some useful questions are:

1. What skills are important for your students to learn?
   The response may range from learning the tai chi form and principles, to the ability to perform certain techniques. Although there is no right or wrong answer, this question gives insight into whether the teacher's delivery mode is teacher or student centered.

2. What is your student population?
   Knowing the age group, gender, and health condition of the students in a class gives a sense of the patient's comfort level with those class participants. If the patient prefers a younger group, then a class composed of older participants may not be suitable. The teaching methods are also likely to reflect the age group.

3. How do you structure your class activities?

   Although tai chi class activities typically involve stepping and standing movements, more teachers are offering chair tai chi or a combination of standing and chair practice. A teacher's flexibility to adapt movements and class activities according to beginners' needs prevents unnecessary physical tension, fatigue, discomfort, or pain.

4. How do you teach?

   This is a broad question. Does the teacher focus on participants' learning, reflection, and experimentation? Is learning the tai chi form the foremost teaching objective? Does the teacher provide room for individuality? How able is the teacher to demonstrate the applications of the tai chi principles? How does the teacher facilitate understanding of the body and its natural movements or adapt the class to participants' specific needs?

5. What participation options are available?

   Participating in a skill-based introductory tai chi class generally serves the needs of most beginners. However, if the patient has complex or specific health conditions, it may be beneficial to build fundamental skills such as body awareness during several private sessions with the teacher before participating in a group-based class. For patients with limited resources, a teacher may refer them to free or low-fee tai chi programs that a community center or library offers.

6. Do you foresee learning challenges with the patient's limitations?

   Many tai chi teachers are unfamiliar with or uninterested in with teaching outside of the realm of the tai chi form and skill. For patients who are concerned with their limitations, care is warranted to select a teacher who:

   - Recommends an appropriate class if class options are available
   - Is able to balance teaching the class and meeting the patient's needs[87]
   - Encourages the application of tai chi concepts to daily functions
   - Offers private lessons for the patient's conditions or limitations
   - Values and supports individual growth and development[87]
   - Refers to helpful resources

Safety concepts

Tai chi is a safe practice because it emphasizes alignment in dynamic and coordinated movement. These slow and deliberate movements increase body awareness, how one moves, and how to optimally move to minimize the risk of injury. However, it is important for beginners to observe some precautions for a healthy and safe learning experience and to discuss their specific limitations or conditions with their teachers.

Decreased Overall Range of Motion

People's movement qualities change over time because of aging, injuries, illness, and chronic pain. Natural movements may become effortful, rigid, and less coordinated, leading to forming a new movement norm. A simple movement of lifting the arms to shoulder level could turn into complicated engagement of different parts of the trunk, such as elevated shoulders, backward upper back leaning, locked elbows and wrists, stiff neck, rigid chest, and holding the breath. Performing 75% or less of the normal range of movement initially may prevent unwarranted fatigue, stiffness, and potential risk of injury.

Attend to Rotational Movements

The waist and hip flexors, the kua, direct upper body movements. Keeping the waist and hip flexors in a relaxed and flexible state in dynamic motion can be challenging initially. Sedentary lifestyle, physical structure, and health conditions often stifle the connection and coordination of these parts of the body. As a result, turning the waist for beginners frequently triggers shoulder, head, or hip-directed rotation, which increases the risk of injuring the back and knees. Learning to identify how the waist and hip flexors turn in a chair and gradually easing into standing and dynamic positions keeps the practice safe and pleasant.

Slow down and Pause

This instruction sounds obvious but it is often challenging for beginners. To incorporate a natural breathing pattern and relaxed state into every step, push, and turn initially requires conscious efforts. This meditative process helps quiet the mind and brings clarity to learning moving with ease. Most importantly, it reduces the risk of injury during practice and in daily activities.

Honor Your Limitations

Everyone has limitations. Advise patients to inform the teacher of movement challenges and encourage the patients to listen to their bodies. Signs of knee locking, chest and shoulder stiffness, and breath holding suggest the body is under stress. Easing the movement effort or performing only a portion of the full movement generally helps prevent hyperextension and reduce unnecessary stress and frustration.

Home practice

Keep it enjoyable and playful. Focus on tai chi principles and experiment with applying them to daily activities. Allow ample time to process and internalize the sensation and relationship of effortless movement and natural body movement. Of utmost importance for patients with chronic health conditions, practicing small sections and avoiding fixation on accuracy avoids frustration and increases self-confidence and self-efficacy.

Perspectives on video use

Videos are useful educational tools. However, patients are likely to gain minimal health benefits from following a tai chi video. Inadvertently, learning from videos without hands-on instruction from a tai chi teacher could potentially lead to undesirable outcomes such as overexertion, rigidity, and misunderstanding of important safety and theoretic concepts, or result in an injury. Some potential advantages and disadvantages of video use for beginners without a tai chi teacher's guidance or instruction are listed here:

Potential advantages of video

- Accessible
- Information gathering
- Isolated movement demonstrations
- Tai chi form demonstrations
- Reinforce class learning (under a teacher's video recommendation)

Potential disadvantages

- Confusing movement directions and concept relationships
- Poor depth perception
- Increased cognitive load and reduced attention to self (movement and state)
- Inadequate understanding of movement appropriateness and adaptations
- Interpret movements from personal experiences rather than from the tai chi lens

Perspectives on tele tai chi classes

Traditional face-to-face tai chi group or private offerings potentially limit accessibility for community dwellers and patients with transportation and distance challenges. Nevertheless, the recent advent of video conferencing technology and increased demand for telemedicine have prompted the development of tele tai chi class and private sessions for the broader community and patients. Much research is warranted to assess the dynamics, outcomes, and value of this innovative platform for tai chi learning and teaching.

Authors' note: this article was being completed during the 2019 to 2020 COVID-19 pandemic. Many complementary and alternative classes, including mindfulness meditation and movement classes such as Yoga and tai chi offered by private, community, and other organizations, quickly migrated to on-line and remote offerings. The authors anticipate new best-practice and evidence-based protocols will emerge from alternative class formats mandated by social distancing guidelines.

UNITED STATES POSTAL SERVICE ®
Statement of Ownership, Management, and Circulation
(All Periodicals Publications Except Requester Publications)

1. Publication Title	2. Publication Number	3. Filing Date
NURSING CLINICS OF NORTH AMERICA	598 – 960	9/18/2020

4. Issue Frequency	5. Number of Issues Published Annually	6. Annual Subscription Price
MAR, JUN, SEP, DEC	4	$163.00

7. Complete Mailing Address of Known Office of Publication (Not printer) (Street, city, county, state, and ZIP+4®)

ELSEVIER INC.
230 Park Avenue, Suite 800
New York, NY 10169

Contact Person
Malathi Samayan

Telephone (Include area code)
91-44-4299-4507

8. Complete Mailing Address of Headquarters or General Business Office of Publisher (Not printer)

ELSEVIER INC.
230 Park Avenue, Suite 800
New York, NY 10169

9. Full Names and Complete Mailing Addresses of Publisher, Editor, and Managing Editor (Do not leave blank)

Publisher (Name and complete mailing address)

DOLORES MELONI, ELSEVIER INC.
1600 JOHN F KENNEDY BLVD. SUITE 1800
PHILADELPHIA, PA 19103-2899

Editor (Name and complete mailing address)

KERRY HOLLAND, ELSEVIER INC.
1600 JOHN F KENNEDY BLVD. SUITE 1800
PHILADELPHIA, PA 19103-2899

Managing Editor (Name and complete mailing address)

PATRICK MANLEY, ELSEVIER INC.
1600 JOHN F KENNEDY BLVD. SUITE 1800
PHILADELPHIA, PA 19103-2899

10. Owner (Do not leave blank. If the publication is owned by a corporation, give the name and address of the corporation immediately followed by the names and addresses of all stockholders owning or holding 1 percent or more of the total amount of stock. If not owned by a corporation, give the names and addresses of the individual owners. If owned by a partnership or other unincorporated firm, give its name and address as well as those of each individual owner. If the publication is published by a nonprofit organization, give its name and address.)

Full Name	Complete Mailing Address
WHOLLY OWNED SUBSIDIARY OF REED/ELSEVIER, US HOLDINGS	1600 JOHN F KENNEDY BLVD. SUITE 1800 PHILADELPHIA, PA 19103-2899

11. Known Bondholders, Mortgagees, and Other Security Holders Owning or Holding 1 Percent or More of Total Amount of Bonds, Mortgages, or Other Securities. If none, check box ► ☐ None

Full Name	Complete Mailing Address
N/A	

12. Tax Status (For completion by nonprofit organizations authorized to mail at nonprofit rates) (Check one)
The purpose, function, and nonprofit status of this organization and the exempt status for federal income tax purposes:

☒ Has Not Changed During Preceding 12 Months
☐ Has Changed During Preceding 12 Months (Publisher must submit explanation of change with this statement)

PS Form **3526**, July 2014 (Page 1 of 4 (see instructions page 4)) PSN: 7530-01-000-9931 PRIVACY NOTICE: See our privacy policy on www.usps.com.

---

13. Publication Title		14. Issue Date for Circulation Data Below
NURSING CLINICS OF NORTH AMERICA		JUNE 2020

15. Extent and Nature of Circulation			Average No. Copies Each Issue During Preceding 12 Months	No. Copies of Single Issue Published Nearest to Filing Date
a. Total Number of Copies (Net press run)			401	335
b. Paid Circulation (By Mail and Outside the Mail)	(1)	Mailed Outside-County Paid Subscriptions Stated on PS Form 3541 (Include paid distribution above nominal rate, advertiser's proof copies, and exchange copies)	281	230
	(2)	Mailed In-County Paid Subscriptions Stated on PS Form 3541 (Include paid distribution above nominal rate, advertiser's proof copies, and exchange copies)	0	0
	(3)	Paid Distribution Outside the Mails Including Sales Through Dealers and Carriers, Street Vendors, Counter Sales, and Other Paid Distribution Outside USPS®	83	75
	(4)	Paid Distribution by Other Classes of Mail Through the USPS (e.g. First-Class Mail®)	0	0
c. Total Paid Distribution (Sum of 15b (1), (2), (3), and (4))			364	305
d. Free or Nominal Rate Distribution (By Mail and Outside the Mail)	(1)	Free or Nominal Rate Outside-County Copies included on PS Form 3541	37	30
	(2)	Free or Nominal Rate In-County Copies included on PS Form 3541	0	0
	(3)	Free or Nominal Rate Copies Mailed at Other Classes Through the USPS (e.g. First-Class Mail)	0	0
	(4)	Free or Nominal Rate Distribution Outside the Mail (Carriers or other means)	37	30
e. Total Free or Nominal Rate Distribution (Sum of 15d (1), (2), (3) and (4))			37	30
f. Total Distribution (Sum of 15c and 15e)			401	335
g. Copies not Distributed (See Instructions to Publishers #4 (page #3))			0	0
h. Total (Sum of 15f and g)			401	335
i. Percent Paid (15c divided by 15f times 100)			90.7%	91.04%

* If you are claiming electronic copies, go to line 16 on page 3. If you are not claiming electronic copies, skip to line 17 on page 3.

UNITED STATES POSTAL SERVICE ®
Statement of Ownership, Management, and Circulation
(All Periodicals Publications Except Requester Publications)

16. Electronic Copy Circulation	Average No. Copies Each Issue During Preceding 12 Months	No. Copies of Single Issue Published Nearest to Filing Date
a. Paid Electronic Copies		
b. Total Paid Print Copies (Line 15c) + Paid Electronic Copies (Line 16a)		
c. Total Print Distribution (Line 15f) + Paid Electronic Copies (Line 16a)		
d. Percent Paid (Both Print & Electronic Copies) (16b divided by 16c × 100)		

☒ I certify that 50% of all my distributed copies (electronic and print) are paid above a nominal price.

17. Publication of Statement of Ownership

☒ If the publication is a general publication, publication of this statement is required. Will be printed in the DECEMBER 2020 issue of this publication.

☐ Publication not required.

18. Signature and Title of Editor, Publisher, Business Manager, or Owner	Date
Malathi Samayan - Distribution Controller *Malathi Samayan*	9/18/2020

I certify that all information furnished on this form is true and complete. I understand that anyone who furnishes false or misleading information on this form or who omits material or information requested on the form may be subject to criminal sanctions (including fines and imprisonment) and/or civil sanctions (including civil penalties).

PS Form **3526**, July 2014 (Page 3 of 4) PRIVACY NOTICE: See our privacy policy on www.usps.com

Moving?

Make sure your subscription moves with you!

To notify us of your new address, find your **Clinics Account Number** (located on your mailing label above your name), and contact customer service at:

Email: **journalscustomerservice-usa@elsevier.com**

800-654-2452 (subscribers in the U.S. & Canada)
314-447-8871 (subscribers outside of the U.S. & Canada)

Fax number: 314-447-8029

Elsevier Health Sciences Division
Subscription Customer Service
3251 Riverport Lane
Maryland Heights, MO 63043

*To ensure uninterrupted delivery of your subscription, please notify us at least 4 weeks in advance of move.

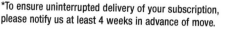

Printed and bound by CPI Group (UK) Ltd, Croydon, CR0 4YY

03/10/2024

01040483-0015